Relief

At-Home, Drug-Free Solutions to Neck, Shoulder & Headache Pain

Dr. Michael Ho

DRTV Asia Ltd.
Niagara Falls, New York

Published by drtv asia limited

Library of Congress Catalog Card Number 2006905969

Relief At-Home, Drug-Free Solutions to Neck, Shoulder & Headache Pain / Dr. Michael Ho

ISBN 0-9787126-1-7

Address for orders:
DRTV Asia Ltd., 1711 Cudaback Avenue Unit #216,
Niagara Falls, New York 14303
Phone 1-877-374-6669
Fax (905) 471-2608
Email drho@drhonow.com
Website http://www.NeckComforter.com

PRINTED IN CHINA

Table of Contents

Introduction

As someone showing an interest in this book, it's likely that you or someone you know suffers from headaches, neck pain or shoulder pain – three of the most common conditions I have treated during my nineteen years of practice as a chiropractor and acupuncturist. You may have noticed that it seems quite ordinary for people to make the offhand comments that they have migraine headaches, carpal tunnel syndrome, a chronically sore shoulder or that they frequently awaken with a stiff neck. An unfortunate truth about these conditions is that they usually recur, sometimes repeatedly over the years, and are so seldom treated successfully by the conventional medical system that the sufferer simply resigns him- or herself to a lifetime of pain.

If you find yourself among the group I just described, you're not alone. The statistics on muscular pain conditions are alarming: they are the number one cause of worker absenteeism in the US and cost upwards of $60 billion annually to treat. Typically all the money spent on medical treatment does not produce results that are as successful as the body's own ability to heal, meaning most of these billions are simply wasted. It has been estimated that close to 80 percent of North Americans have suffered or suffer regularly from one or more of these pain disorders. Among the thousands of patients I treat in my practice, a disproportionately large number complain of varying forms of head, neck, shoulder and limb pain. For every patient seeking treatment, however, there are many who are not, either because they lack the time, are adopting a "wait and see" approach to their pain, lack the insurance or financial resources, or are simply cynical about the effectiveness of treatment. It is for both my regular patients and those whom I will never meet that I have written this book. It is my single mission to help you rid yourself of pain for good – without surgery, symptom-masking medications, time-consuming rituals or other disruptions to your life.

Even if you suffer from a disorder that produces ongoing muscular spasm and chronic pain such as fibromyalgia, *Dr. Ho's Hands-On Solutions to Neck, Shoulder and Headache Problems* can help ease your discomfort, no matter your physical condition, age or level of fitness, and put you on the path to a happier and more productive life. Through education and the methods of self-treatment provided herein, you can relieve your pain without the ceaseless appointments and wasted money so many experience using today's healthcare system, and with true and lasting results.

This concise book provides simple solutions for even the worst conditions, ends the mystery of chronic pain and its causes, and offers sound advice on medication, lifestyle, body mechanics and the need for integrated physical and emotional support to help you avoid injury and suffering – now and for the rest of your life.

Both from my own experience, and from the experiences of the thousands of patients who have walked through my doors, I know how plaguing pain like migraines, arthritis or chronic muscle stiffness can be. They can force you to take bed rest, make you use sick leave, or at the very least substantially cut into your production at the workplace. At home, you may find that you lack the energy to properly care for or interact with your family, perform routine tasks and simply to be your normal loveable self. Pain, particularly the chronic variety, can make it hard to be social and productive. When suffered over a period longer than a couple weeks, or when experienced repeatedly, pain can lead to depression, isolation and an inability to enjoy life as normal. The goal when faced with recurrent neck, shoulder or headache problems is to treat the source of the pain, avoid unnecessary treatments that don't address the root problem (and can lead to side effects of their own) and learn how to keep these problems from returning.

With the aid of *Dr. Ho's Hands-On Solutions to Neck, Shoulder and Headache Problems,* you'll learn how to communicate the right information to your doctor during your limited appointment time, improve your treatment and alleviate much of your doctor's guesswork. This book will also help you to recognize the source of your pain and treat it appropriately yourself, so that you can limit your trips to the doctor, and help prevent pain episodes in the future. Whether your condition is something like simple neck stiffness to a more serious one like fibromyalgia, your pain can be treated and controlled, and in many cases eliminated for good. But first, let's discuss the cornerstone of your treatment, the understanding of what causes your headache, neck or shoulder pain in the first place. You may be surprised.

CHAPTER ONE

What's Causing My Pain

Two questions my patients commonly have are: *Why does it seem that more people suffer from head, neck and shoulder pain than ever before?* and *Why hasn't my MD been able to cure my pain?* Let me address both of those questions before we go any further, for they are the basis of this book and a major aspect of my practice.

I agree that the numbers of people suffering from these pain conditions are increasing, and at a perplexing rate. Many of my patients remark that they don't recall their parents or other relatives complaining of such maladies years ago – they might remember their mother having an occasional headache, but those memories seldom include her having spent the day in bed in a dark room, completely incapacitated. Few people I've interviewed remember any adult from their childhood having tendinitis in his or her hands. Didn't people suffer from these conditions forty years ago? Certainly they did, but not in the numbers that we see today. And the natural question in response is: *Why?*

There are many possible answers. One is that productivity in our part of the world is more intense than ever before – we work longer hours, produce more per hour and have more demands placed on us than our parents or grandparents did. The average

North American now works eighty hours more per year than was the norm fifty years ago. For most employees, regular, substantial breaks are a thing of the past – ten minutes every few hours must do, with thirty to sixty minutes for a lunch that sometimes gets consumed at a desk or in a car. The survival of most families now requires both parents (or a single parent) to work outside the home, which translates to increased work for everyone concerned, with home duties an additional burden after long hours on the job. People have less time to relax, to enjoy leisure activities and to engage in the types of exercise that were once considered a normal part of life, like taking a stroll or gardening – simple acts that keep the body and mind loose and fluid.

Our physical and emotional stressors are immense, our time is tapped and there is no end in sight. For many of us the only enjoyable part of the week is the weekend, but even then we find ourselves so exhausted that we spend it collapsed on the couch. From car to desk to car to couch, often with a cellphone cradled against one's neck, is not a healthy way to live, but it has become the norm for many of us. And there in the backs of our minds is that ever-present push to do more, produce more, achieve more. No wonder we're feeling squeezed, both emotionally and physically.

This lifestyle has produced a startling number of working people who suffer from neck- and shoulder-related problems, beginning as early as age thirty. Too much stationary or repetitive work that forces people into bad postures and allows them few breaks causes muscles to become contracted and, over time, to actually *harden*. I often hear, "Oh, Doc, my neck and shoulders feel like rocks." This comment indicates a serious problem that patients are noticing themselves: their muscles are in a state of constant contraction.

Frequently, this begins to feel normal to people: knots in the upper back where the muscles meet the neck, stiffness in the neck itself, pain in a wrist or elbow becomes just another part of the day. But in order to demonstrate what muscles *should* feel like, let's look at an example of a muscle that in most people remains in a healthy state: the biceps. The biceps are the muscles on the inside of your upper arm, the ones you flex when you're showing off. If you take your relaxed left biceps muscle and squeeze it with your right hand, you'll notice that it's smooth and supple – no knots, no rigidity. This is what a healthy muscle feels like, firm but not tight. If, however, you held a five-pound weight absolutely still in your right hand with your elbow bent for even half an hour every day for a week, you'd notice that your right biceps would be tight because you've taught it to stay contracted. Imagine if you held that weight for months, even years: this muscle would become rock hard, even at rest. Healthy muscle is hard when flexed and firm but supple when relaxed – unhealthy muscle never relaxes and may be simultaneously weak *and* hard, stiff, lacking movement, and sore to the touch or when stretched, because it has become riddled with scar tissue. And this from only five pounds, half the weight of the average head.

So now you have an idea of what's been happening to your neck – it constantly supports weight and gets little rest or proper exercise. This ongoing *isometric contraction*, as described in the biceps example, invites muscle stiffness and pain. And life as we now know it creates a perfect environment for neck dysfunction.

Consider, too, the many repetitive occupational activities that may cause people pain: hunching in front of a computer; bending over to assemble something in a factory; taking calls on a hand-held phone instead of a headset; driving for hours a day. Add to these everyday functions the stress of household commitments like cooking, looking after kids and worrying about your finances and you have a recipe for agony.

The biceps muscles in the above example cause few problems.

Why? They are muscles that inherently get treated well, even by sedentary people. Even a "couch potato" uses his biceps every day, from brushing his teeth to opening the fridge to lifting a glass to his lips. They get stretched regularly because when not in use they are well-extended along our sides. And they get the complete rest they need to repair everyday damage during sleep, when they are not used at all. Thus, except for sustaining random injuries or being used in sports that require their overuse, the biceps are typically muscles that are so problem-free that we completely forget about them.

The neck, however, isn't so lucky. Even at rest, our necks find themselves trying to establish balance for our heads – often on pillows that force us into postures that tuck the chin downward, stressing the posterior neck muscles all night long. Or worse, we sleep on our bellies with our heads cranked to one side, causing even more neck strain. If you sleep on your belly, you may notice you prefer to place your head to one side over the other. The result: one side of your neck is strained, the other is in a constant state of muscle contraction.

The shoulder is affected by the mistreatment of the neck because the peripheral nerves that run to the shoulder get their information directly from the central nervous system of the spinal cord. And the top of the spinal cord is situated where? You guessed it, within the neck. So, the twenty-four-hours-a-day beating your neck absorbs has influence on your shoulders, your arms, your upper back, your head – any area that gets its information from the cranial nerves that live in utmost portion of the spinal cord. The constant abuse causes the neck and shoulder muscles to become harder and shorter. As this happens, your range of motion decreases and suddenly you realize, "Gee, I can't turn my head as far as I used to be able to." Actually, this development has progressed steadily over time and will continue to get worse if you don't take steps now to treat it.

In my practice one of the first tests I perform on patients is to measure their range of movement. I find that from age thirty onward most adults have lost anywhere from twenty to eighty percent of their normal range of motion and they frequently don't even know it. They may not be in any pain, but they can't move their necks as well as they could the year before, or the year before that.

The unfortunate fact about joints is that when they're not allowed to move fully on a regular basis, they start to deteriorate faster than normal. Movement initiates a lubricating fluid within the joints to wash over the cartilage and keep them healthy, but once your body experiences a reduction in motion it deprives the joints of natural nourishment and washing. Once a joint is deprived long enough, its degeneration can lead to related conditions like arthritis, even in younger people. In fact, the majority of patients I see who complain of neck pain and headaches produce X-rays showing some stage of arthritis – even people in their thirties who report no incidents that might explain its early onset. This is a disturbing trend indeed. I can only conclude that these early arthritic conditions are the direct result of everyday strain on neck and shoulder muscles.

To give you an example, I recently treated an eighty-year-old mother and her forty-year-old daughter, both of whom had been involved in a car accident. The mother had never had any neck problems in the past, but the daughter reported that she'd had neck stiffness for years. After X-raying both, I found that the eighty-year-old mother showed no degeneration of her joints: they were smooth, her discs were well-rounded and situated perfectly between the vertebrae and her spine was in correct alignment. However, her forty-year-old daughter's discs showed significant deterioration: they had changed shape and become narrow. Her joints were rough and arthritic and my analysis of her X-ray indicated that degeneration had begun in her twenties. Upon questioning her, I discovered that the daughter had been involved in two previous car accidents, one fifteen years before and another eight years ago. In all three accident cases, her car was rear-ended by another while she was stopped at a red light. Our interview also revealed that the daughter worked long hours doing computer-related work that she found quite stressful and that she engaged in no regular exercise program. The multiple injuries combined with a sedentary lifestyle had caused her neck and shoulder muscles to become tense and shortened. Those constantly contracted muscles in turn created a loss of joint movement in her neck that led to premature degeneration of her cervical discs.

The elderly mother, on the other hand, had been lucky enough never to have been in a car accident until the one that brought her into my clinic. During most of her life she'd been a stay-at-home mom whose work looking after three children involved duties that kept her naturally active and mobile. The physical demands of tending to domestic work, combined with her accident-free history, had kept her muscles and joints in shape and her discs free of measurable degeneration.

The truth about disc degeneration, known as *osteoarthritis*, is that it can come at almost any age, and is caused by the ongoing dysfunction of the neck and spine. This dysfunction causes a breakdown of the cartilage that protects and cushions the joints. Continued degeneration of the cartilage can actually allow the bones that it previously protected to rub against each other and create serious discomfort.

Osteoarthritis can strike anyone whose muscles tighten so much that they disallow the spine from working correctly and limits his or her range of motion. Degenerative arthritic change is irreversible and can start to show itself in as little as *five years* of whatever caused its onset, whether it was an accident or recurrent abuse.

Sarah is a patient who demonstrates a classic scenario I see regularly at my pain clinic. She came to me with serious neck pain that radiated into her head. She was understandably alarmed and said that the pain "came out of nowhere, Doc. I just woke up the other day and there it was." But her X-rays showed arthritic changes indicating the problem had begun many years before, long before she had symptoms. I suggested that we look over her history. "Have you had any injuries, even a long time ago?" I asked. "Did you fall down, have a car accident, get hit, anything?" Upon thinking about it, she revealed that she'd had a simple "fender-bender" just over five years ago. Her neck had felt a little stiff for a couple of weeks afterward and then it "just seemed to go away." This is exactly this kind of minor injury that typically never goes away completely, and triggers subtle muscle tension that starts to cut down a person's range of motion. It is so subtle that it goes unnoticed or ignored for years and then gets the attention it deserves only years later when it creates the pain signalling a degenerative arthritic change.

To prevent this debilitating development, it's crucial to regularly loosen the neck and shoulder muscles. Sounds simple enough, right? This simple muscular relaxation restores the range of motion of the upper joints of the spine, and can be achieved through massage to increase circulation, gentle stretching to increase movement, and regular exercise to maintain and increase muscular strength, encourage washing of the cartilage in our joints and enhance our ability to rest. Now some of you may think of the word *exercise* with the same affection that you'd view a draft notice. But I'm not talking about gruelling exercise – I'm suggesting exercise so simple that is should be considered *normal and necessary movement*.

As an example of this premise let's look at your elbow. Most of us have healthy elbows that can move in a full range; you can probably bend and straighten your arm without any problem. But imagine placing your elbow in a hard cast, one that allows your elbow no movement, for six months. Once I cut off the cast and take an X-ray of your formerly healthy elbow, we would very likely find some early degenerative changes in it. The long and short of it is: movement encourages health, inactivity invites dysfunction.

A case of zero movement, of course, is extreme, but the range of motion many people currently experience in a day is frighteningly close to the example. You may jog, you may eat right, but when is the last time you did any exercise or even deliberate movement of your neck? The neck, in spite of its importance, is easy to ignore, and degenerative changes in it are subtle and take place over enough years that most people don't realize anything is happening until they wake up one day and realize suddenly that their necks don't move well. Few would associate it with hours at a desk or time spent cradling a phone, or with an accident that happened years ago and left no apparent problems, but these are exactly the types of things that can cause ongoing problems.

Once these pain conditions crop up, we are perplexed and forced suddenly to seek medical attention. We go to our doctors and then on to specialists, but we still haven't put together what caused the problem to begin with, and typically the professionals we see seem as clueless as we are. They test, they poke at our sore spots and then we leave hoping for the best, but too often we get little or no relief. Which brings us to the next question patients ask: *Why hasn't my MD been able to cure my pain?*

The reasons why standard medicine is so often ineffective in treating common pain conditions are several and most are probably not the direct fault of your doctor. Most **MDS**, including those who specialize in the treatment of the muscles, nerves and bones, are very hard-working, diligent people who have found themselves caught in the maze of managed care, and they find it as frustrating as you do. They are required to see a requisite number of people a day, are instructed to spend no more than a few minutes with each and are under great pressure to move along through the roster of patients as quickly as possible and prescribe a minimum course of treatment to limit costs. MDS treat a vast variety of ailments and injuries every day, from athlete's foot to concussions, and very few have the time or inclination to focus on something as specific as the treatment of pain disorders – it is but one tiny segment of what they've learned to do in the course of their education. Most have been trained to first investigate possible pathology and infection, which is good medicine, but when neither of those situations turns up, they often decide the disorder isn't serious and fail to give it their full attention, which is bad medicine. To be frank, the treatment of pain is usually an ongoing process, one the healthcare establishment places very low on its list of priorities and one that can be potentially expensive to treat. It may be one reason why so little attention is paid to musculoskeletal medicine in the education of even *orthopedists*, doctors specializing in disorders of the bones and muscles. A study of recent medical school graduates by the University School of Medicine, Philadelphia, Pennsylvania produced these findings:

> *According to [a basic competency examination], 82 percent of the examinees failed to demonstrate basic competency in musculoskeletal medicine. It is therefore reasonable to conclude that medical school preparation in musculoskeletal medicine is inadequate.*[1]

This is a disturbing finding, considering these are the specialists

[1]From *Journal of Bone and Joint Surgery* (Amer) 2002; 84-A (4) Apr: 604 608; Freedman, Bernstein.

many of us see in the course of our pain treatment. The end result is that patients receive insufficient care because the diagnosis and treatment of pain disorders has proven to be one of the major failings of the modern healthcare system.

Another reason for this failing, however, is the impatience of patients. The same demand by patients for instant gratification that saw doctors erroneously prescribing antibiotics for viruses during the eighties and nineties, has generated the over-prescription of pain medications to people whose pain could be better treated through therapy, exercise and simple lifestyle changes. For example, I know a man in his thirties who has undergone a serious operation for chronic back pain and is contemplating another that would require additional months away from work and time spent convalescing. Yet he has ignored any suggestion that he adopt a regular pattern of exercise to remedy his problem and prevent recurrences in the future. His attitude toward his pain condition is that a doctor should fix it immediately and that he bears no role in this own recovery. One of the missions of this book is to help you to understand how to assist your healthcare provider so that he or she can properly diagnose and treat your pain disorder, as well as enable you to treat it yourself at home and prevent its return. How do I know how to do this? Simple. I've learned it from my patients.

For many people, the idea of being labeled a "patient" is a horrifying thing; it sounds like circumstances are spinning outside their control. The truth is, the more control you take over your own care, the better your result and the less money and time you will spend on it. This book is not a substitute for appropriate healthcare, but rather an important addition to it. Only a *qualified healthcare practitioner* can diagnose any medical condition and it is important to have your doctor perform the proper diagnostic examination before your treatment begins, to rule out less common but very serious possible causes of headaches and neck and shoulder pain, such as meningitis and even heart disease.

Pain in the Neck

Over my many years as a chiropractor and an acupuncturist, I've treated countless patients with headaches and neck, shoulder, arm and hand pain. People describe how their migraines keep them up at night, how their repetitive stress injuries won't go away, that their muscles ache as if they were on fire. Most have tried the conventional medicine route and have left with a bottle of pills, still in pain and without any clue as to the actual reason for their condition.

I'm going to suggest a cause that will sound so simple that you may be skeptical of it: the source of almost all migraine headache, neck and shoulder pain is contracted muscles and the inflammation of associated nerves in the neck. Yes, the neck – the small structure that supports the ten-pound globe of your head and encases the top part of your spine, along with a very complicated system of nerves – is the hub of most of your pain problems.

How can muscles in your neck cause tenosynovitis of the thumb or a blinding ache in your temples? It is perhaps a design flaw of the human body, at least for today's lifestyle needs, that this relatively puny and very vulnerable area is so vital; it is the exit point of the eight pairs of nerves that supply the head, neck, upper back, shoulders, arms and hands. If the muscles supporting your neck are in a state of unremitting contraction, they will cause great irritation to the nerves that supply those muscles, and pain and degeneration will result – not only in your neck, but in the tendons of your shoulder, the nerves that travel from your neck to your head, even those that run through your shoulders down to your arms and hands. Nineteen years of treating patients have demonstrated time and again that migraine headache, dizziness, tennis elbow, carpal tunnel syndrome, arthritis of the hands and many other very common maladies have their root cause in contracted muscles in the neck. A stiff neck is more than an annoyance, it is usually the sign that something is wrong and, left untreated, it will get worse over time.

The neck has two contributing factors to its vulnerability: one, it is very small relative to its importance and two, it suffers mightily from what I call the "Abuse of Disuse." No part of the body contributes more greatly to every aspect of upper body movement than the neck – even at rest it is supporting the position of your head – and yet none is so mistreated. So for many of us problems start to crop up when we hit our thirties, at a time when we are still young enough to feel unbreakable, but our bodies are beginning to succumb to the abuse and neglect of our youth. And the abuse and neglect begin early, sometimes from the moment of birth.

Even a smooth, uncomplicated delivery through the birth canal exerts a tractional force of about ninety pounds on a baby's tiny, fragile neck. And if there is any complication, that force is substantially greater and there is a strong possibility that minor neck injuries can be sustained. We see it with a condition called *torticollis,* also known as wry neck, in which an infant has a muscle spasm so severe that it can't turn its neck and is stuck with it turned to one side. Often parents bring babies with wry neck to my clinic to receive instructions on how to massage and very gently stretch the neck to restore movement. But for every parent who learns how to do this, the vast majority do not and the process of chronic neck stiffness has begun. Most parents may not even be aware that anything is wrong – something so minor can easily go unnoticed even by health professionals, and get incrementally worse over time.

As infants become toddlers, the majority will have minor accidents learning to navigate their way across the floor, up the stairs, onto furniture. If you can think of a child who hasn't once fallen on his head or banged his chin against a hard object, then you'd better write to Guinness! Falls from swing sets, trees, blows from sports, tripping while running – you name it – are all sources of minor trauma. Any kid who has ever bounced a soccer ball off his or her head has borne substantial added weight and blunt force to the neck. Once they begin school, children spend hours sitting at desks that may be ill-sized for them, hunched over books and paperwork, and at angles where they're forced to look at a chalkboard in an awkward position. Once the school bell rings many swing heavy book bags over one shoulder and return home to sit hunched in front of the TV for extended periods, chins on hands, and you have the foundation of neck problems awaiting them as they approach middle age.

Children, resilient beings that they are, don't usually notice pain or, if they do, are inclined to ignore it. As we grow older, our bad body mechanics have already become ingrained as habits. So, long before we enter the workaday world of sitting for long hours at a desk and/or in a car – or are subjected to movements that get repeated over and over such as typing, hammering, kneading dough, etc. – bad posture, immobility, misuse and disuse of the neck have already begun to take their toll. From there things get worse, and our range of motion becomes compromised. Once that happens our likelihood of injury, even without a specific triggering event, becomes great.

Naturally we can't step back in time and reverse all the abuse that our necks may have encountered during the course of our lives. But we can educate ourselves on the roots and causes of neck stiffness, and use our knowledge to assist our healthcare providers in administering correct treatment, help rid ourselves of pain at home, and develop healthy body mechanics to help prevent future problems. The beginning of the process is understanding the conditions that make us vulnerable to neck dysfunction and its related pain syndromes.

Is a Stiff Neck a Serious Problem?

Anything that puts you in pain and diminishes your capacity to function and enjoy life should be considered serious, whatever its cause. By the time most people come to me for chiropractic and/or acupuncture treatment, they are in pain. After all, by the nature of my practice, I am a pain doctor: people see me for relief and to help them facilitate and maintain movement, not for a suspicious mole or an ingrown toenail or the myriad other problems that might take them to their regular **MDS**. And most have tried conventional medicine and are using chiropractic/acupuncture as a part of their therapy or because other therapies have failed them. For many patients, what brings them in is a calamity, commonly an auto accident, where they sustained whiplash or some other tangible injury. Many seem indifferent when I ask if they've had years of neck stiffness in the morning or limited range of movement as if they think it is irrelevant to their present injury. But in fact those ignored symptoms have set the stage for their suffering and most should have sought treatment long before they got rear-ended at a stoplight. More than any other cause, chronic muscle tension is the source of pain from many different common conditions. In order to better understand why this happens, let's take a closer look at the basic anatomy of the body and how it enables pain to occur.

A Guide to Muscles, Nerves, Blood Vessels and Joints

Let's define the tissues and how muscle tension causes pain:

1. **Muscles** – *A group of fibres that contract and relax to facilitate movement. When muscles contract, the length of the muscle fibres becomes shorter; when they are relaxed, they lengthen. The nerves supplying the muscle fibres control the amount of muscle contraction. When nerves become hyperactive they can cause muscles to remain contracted indefinitely.*

2. **Tendons** – *These elastic tissues, located at both ends of the muscle fibres, attach muscle to bone. The amount of tensile strain on the tendon depends on the contraction and length of the muscle. Contracted muscles will cause extra strain on the associated tendon(s).*

3. **Nerves** – *The soft and sensitive electrical wiring of the body. Signals from the motor nerves give the muscles the electrical power to contract. Sensory nerves receive various stimuli and send these sensations to the spinal cord and brain. Nerve fibres, located beside or inside muscle fibres, conduct electrical impulses through the body and are very sensitive to pressure. Constant pressure placed on nerves by contracted muscles will cause pain, numbness and dysfunction.*

4. **Joints** – *The articulating surface between two moving bones. The cartilage surface of the joints is smooth and lubricated to allow full motion. Full range of movement is necessary to keep the joint cartilage well-lubricated and healthy. Contracted muscles will decrease joint movement.*

5. **Arteries and Veins** – *The tubes inside and around muscle*

fibres that take blood to and from the heart and supply the body's tissues and organs. Contracted muscles can constrict these vessels and decrease blood circulation, causing pain to the deprived muscles.

In order to understand how commonly pain conditions like chronic stiffness, migraines, carpal tunnel syndrome and other disorders relate to the contraction of muscles comprising the neck, let's take a brief look at the neck itself.

The Anatomy of the Neck

The neck contains and supports the vital transactions between your head and body, including passages for air and food and major blood vessels and nerves. The neck is made up of a surprising number of muscles and nerves given its size, all of which were engineered for maximum stability and mobility of the head. The muscles of the neck are much more complex than one might think. The front (anterior) and the back (posterior) views of the muscle sets of the neck show two major triangles and multiple smaller triangles, each of which control and support different functions. The anterior muscles control everything from swallowing to tongue movement to speech, and support the neck's lymph nodes. Another muscle system connects the respiratory skeleton to the sternum, which is located all the way down at the centre of your chest. Because the neck also acts as the housing for the upper spinal cord and the vertebral column, it contains the eight sets of nerves that control your head and neck, your diaphragm and the muscles of your shoulders, arms, wrists and hands. In other words, its influence on your body as a whole is massive.

The posterior muscles, those at the back of the neck, have a higher proportion of "slow twitch" muscle fibres than the anteriors, meaning they are more efficient performing functions demanding endurance, such as holding up and balancing your head for extended hours at a time. The act of looking straight up into the sky causes these posterior muscles to contract greatly and absorb weight at an awkward suspension, which is why it so quickly becomes uncomfortable to sustain. On the other hand, these muscles also have unusual demands placed on them when your head is bent slightly forward or off to one side, since the heaviness of your head is no longer supported as well by your spinal column. Think of an ice cream cone being tilted to the side: naturally gravity takes over and beckons the ice cream to topple over the cone onto the ground (which is usually what happens, much to the dismay of your average child). In the case of the neck, the posterior muscles work continuously to keep your head from toppling over, a function so constant that we take it for granted.

This tilted head posture is what most of us adopt in all avenues of our lives. We stand and walk with our heads bowed forward, we sit for long hours working, reading or watching TV with our chins tilted toward our chests or pushed forward off the centre of our spines; we angle our necks to the left or right to support a phone and then at night we compound the problem by sleeping with our heads cranked to one side or angled awkwardly on pillows that are too lofty or lack support. The muscles forming the posterior triangle are almost constantly at work, yet seldom exercised. Over time, repeated minor straining of these neck muscles will cause them to stay tensed. Given our incredible abuses of this prone but incredibly important body part, it is something of a miracle that we can move our heads at all.

By now you may be saying, "Okay, Dr. Ho, I know that I might not treat my neck as well as I should, but why is that causing me to have pain in my elbows and forearms?" This question is a logical one and it brings us to the involvement of the nerves.

We have an impressive system of peripheral nerves in our bodies and they are responsible for allowing us to feel pleasure, temperature, pain and pressure. These nerves tell you when your shoes are too tight or warn you lightning-quick to take your hand off a hot stove. These nerves travel through every part of your body, crossing through, over and under the muscles from which they accept information, and networking that information through the spinal cord to the brain. When a muscle becomes contracted and inflamed due to strain, disease or injury; or deprived of oxygen; or stiff from disuse, the nerves adjacent to it are also affected. When nerves are under constant pressure from compromised muscle tissues they can become chronically irritated and cause pain and stiffness to persist even after the inflammation is gone. For this reason the benefits of non-steroidal anti-inflammatory drugs (**NSAID**s) like Aspirin, ibuprofen (Advil) and naproxen sodium (Aleve) are far more limited than most people believe. While they can be an effective part of treatment during the initial stages of injury by aiding in the reduction of swelling, once the body conquers the inflammation the meds act only to mask the pain and do nothing further to assist the body's natural defences. In the meantime, the medication takes its toll on your internal organs, like the stomach, liver and kidneys. Over time such medications have actually been shown to produce certain pains they are meant to alleviate, such as headaches.

Therefore, the best ways to relieve pain are ones that allow your body's own defences to take over and heal itself. In cases of constant muscular pain not caused by injury or misuse, as with syndromes like fibromyalgia, medication may be necessary to keep pain at bay on especially bad days, but even in those instances their benefits are limited. Before we fully discuss treatment, however, let's move on to the next chapter and really explore the physical causes of pain.

Notes:

The Origins of Pain

There are many possible causes of headaches and neck and shoulder pain – disc degeneration, arthritis, tendinitis, repetitive stress disorder and fibromyalgia, to name a few – all of which result in muscle tension and irritation of the affected ligaments and nerves. Whatever the cause, the ultimate result is pain. Gaining the most from your treatment is easier when you understand how and why your body creates pain in the first place.

How Does Pain Begin?

All the muscles involved in an act of movement will contract and then, ideally, relax again. This is normal muscle function. Problems begin when the muscle contraction is caused by undue stress, the type we often associate with unpleasant or unhealthy conditions: emotional stress, physical trauma, repetitive strain, hormonal imbalance, poor spinal posture, bad diet, or any situation that is uncomfortable for the body. These conditions cause the related muscles to contract and stay contracted, as if the body were in a constant state of alarm. This instinctive muscular reaction is most likely a product of the body's fight or flight reflex

– something is wrong and the body is preparing for battle. If the source of stress is sustained or repeated over time, the nerves will tell the muscles to stay contracted. After a period of prolonged muscle contraction, the tensed muscles will not relax even with rest. Without proper treatment to relax it, the muscle will continue to contract and will eventually cause pain, from mild to excruciating.

How Do Contracted Muscles Cause Pain?

Muscles that remain contracted for extended periods release noxious inflammatory chemicals that irritate the local tissues and cause them to become sore and tender to the touch. With time, even light pressure on these tender points, also called *trigger points,* will cause hypersensitivity.

Without the regular opportunity to relax, contracted muscles become short and inflexible, decreasing movement in the adjacent joints and creating stiffness. Prolonged stiffness in the joint will cause the smooth cartilage surface of the joint to degenerate prematurely and become inflamed, as with arthritis. Continuous degeneration of the joint will make even simple everyday movements like lifting your arm or turning your head wincingly difficult.

Contracted muscles then irritate the nerves located beside or inside the muscle fibres, causing local nerve pain. Pressure on a nerve can also cause something known as "referred pain," in which pain travels a nerve pathway from its source the neck, to an affected area of the head or upper body. The brain is often poor at interpreting the exact location of a pain source when it exists inside the body and instead ascribes it to a convenient nearby location – pain in the heart is interpreted as pain in the shoulder or left arm, and pain in your kidneys can be felt as a terrible burning in your back. Common examples of this phenomenon as it occurs within the neck are tension headaches and arm pain caused by thoracic outlet syndrome.

Muscle tension along the spine can cause many painful conditions, including migraine and tension headaches, fatigue, dizziness and neck pain. Tight muscles in the upper back and posterior area of the neck can cause limited neck mobility, shoulder soreness and rotator cuff injuries. When the nerves that run from the neck to the arms are irritated, they can cause numbness, pain and weakness in any part of the arm, hand and/or shoulder. This irritation can be a direct cause of carpal tunnel syndrome, tennis elbow and other limb maladies.

Spinal Muscle Tension

One of the most dramatic syndromes of muscular tension involves a neurological process of the muscles and nerves along the spine called *segmental facilitation*.

A frustrating fact about the tension of spinal muscles is that it actually perpetuates itself – muscle tension causes more muscle tension, a vicious cycle of misery. This continuous, accumulating tension causes most of the chronic pain I see in my practice. Segmental facilitation involves either a violent muscle spasm, similar to the knee-jerk reflex, or a slower but excessive contraction of muscles along the spine. Often this spasm is caused by work- or accident-related injuries. It can also be invited by something as simple as sleeping with your neck in a bad posture or keeping your head in a forward position for too long a period while performing work that requires your arms to be forward of your body. For reasons I've already described, the modern lifestyle of sitting too long and moving too little primes us for episodes of segmental facilitation: our neck muscles are constantly being strained and our range of neck motion compromised, vastly increasing the likelihood of painful syndromes related to a dysfunctional neck.

But I Got Injured a Long Time Ago. Why Am I Still in Pain?

One of the most trying facts about segmental facilitation is that once the spasm occurs it can become increasingly worse even if you experience no additional stress or stimulation. Muscle tension along the spine places pressure on the nerves located beside and/or inside the contracted muscle fibres. These nerves then become irritated and hyperactive, causing a reflex reaction within the spinal cord that in turn causes hyperactivity in the motor nerves that control muscle contraction. When the motor nerves are overexcited, they cause the already-tense muscles to contract even more, creating a terrible, agonizing cycle. Over time, this chain reaction will produce more muscle tension, pain and stiffness, so that the spasm reaction is triggered by even small amounts of stress – whether emotional or physical.

Recently I met a forty-two year-old woman named Debra who described her experience with this syndrome. She noted that lately she'd been waking up every morning with a stiff neck and severe migraine headaches. During our interview I discovered that she'd had no history of having migraine headaches as a child, but had begun suffering from them only about three years before. They had first been mild and infrequent but had gotten progressively worse to the point where they were diminishing her quality of life. Her general health was excellent, though she reported feeling fatigued even with adequate amounts of sleep. She also noted that about five years before our meeting her car had been rear-ended at a red light. She did not sustain any major injuries but her neck felt tender and tight for a couple of months and she'd had some headaches and mild dizziness for a few weeks afterward. She went to her doctor, who examined her head and neck, ordered X-rays and prescribed anti-inflammatory medication and muscle relaxants. She took the meds for a few weeks, felt better, and presumed that her neck problem was resolved. From time to time, however, she noticed that her neck still felt tense and that she suffered from occasional headaches. When discussing these concerns with her doctor, they both agreed that it was related to her stressful job as a legal assistant. The fact, however, was that Debra, like countless other patients I've treated, was not diagnosed or treated properly. Complete and correct treatment would have eliminated her recurrent headaches, fatigue and stiff neck, even during times when she experienced emotional stress.

Debra's neck muscles were tense and inflamed from the minor whiplash injury she sustained from the car accident. The meds that her doctor prescribed relieved the symptoms, but did not address her abnormally contracted neck muscles and therefore lent nothing to curing the problem. Over time, her muscle tension created a state of adaptation to a new norm, the condition of being tense, and her muscles fought to maintain their contracted state even during rest. Once this process of segmental facilitation was underway, every source of stress – whether physical or emotional – increased Debra's level of the muscular contraction. Eventually the muscle tension increased to a level where the nerves in her upper neck became so irritated that they caused her to experience headaches.

As the muscle tension in her neck increased, so did the frequency, duration and severity of her migraines. Debra's headaches occurred more frequently in the mornings – after a night of motionless sleep allowed her neck muscles to stiffen even more. If her doctor had recognized and diagnosed her as having segmental facilitation, he probably would have prescribed a course of treatment involving deep tissue massage and function-restoring exercises, and included an effective at-home treatment program utilizing *transcutaneous electrical nerve stimulation*, or **TENS**, which I will describe in detail in the "Treatment and Prevention" chapter. Had she received the proper diagnosis and treatment, I am convinced that her recovery would have been faster, more complete and shown a great reduction in her immediate and long-term suffering.

Not only do chronically contracted muscles remain stiff for days, weeks or even months, they can produce any or all of the following symptoms:

Muscular Ache and Pain

Muscles that are clenched from overuse are the most common cause of aches and pain. These contracted muscles release noxious chemicals that irritate surrounding tissues and create an unwelcome burning sensation. "Overuse injuries" run the entire gamut of repetitive stress disorders, any of which can leave the associated muscles irritated and inflamed even though no obvious injury occurred. Examples of overuse injuries include bursitis, tendinitis (including carpal tunnel), shin splints and stress fractures.

Joint Stiffness and Pain

Sore, stiff joints can be caused by injuries and arthritis, but more commonly they are the result of supporting muscles tightening due to lack of movement. Tight muscles prevent the joint from achieving its full range of motion, interfere with proper joint lubrication and nourishment, and cause joint pain and degeneration. A joint that doesn't move properly will degenerate rapidly; even a young person can develop degenerative joint disease or osteoarthritis from long periods of inactivity.

Poor Circulation

The rate of blood flow through veins and arteries depends upon the diameter of the blood vessel, blood pressure and the pressure exerted from outside the blood vessel wall. Tight muscles around a blood vessel will restrict flow and encourage an accumulation within the muscles of noxious chemicals created by the metabolism of lactic acid. The buildup of these waste chemicals increases tension and pain. Poor circulation also decreases the oxygen to muscles and this deprivation in turn can generate spontaneous muscular spasm. When the blood flow remains constricted by action of the autonomic nerves, the abnormal constriction of the muscle tissue persists, sometimes for agonizingly long periods.

Muscles that are deprived of oxygen are not only prone to spasm and pain-producing waste storage, they create trigger points – spots that are painful when pressed or manipulated. Touch the rear sides of your neck from the base of your skull down to your upper back. Are there tender spots? Now trace your fingers outward to your levator scapulae muscles, where you neck meets your shoulder. Do you feel knots that hurt when you apply pressure? These are trigger points, areas where oxygen absorption is limited due to constant tension. They may not always cause noticeable pain, but the goal is to get rid of any tenderness altogether by increasing circulation and oxygen to those areas.

Nerve Pain and Numbness

Nerves that are irritated or pinched can become numb, tingly or painful along the nerve branches. Tight muscles along the spine frequently irritate nerves, and pinched nerves in the neck can cause headaches, neck pain, shoulder pain and radiating aches down the arms into the hands. A nerve under constant pressure from conditions such as a herniated disc or multiple sclerosis can lose its conductivity.

How Do Aggravated Nerves Cause Pain?

Nerves have a powerful influence on our muscles and joints. Generally speaking, there are two types of nerves in the body: one type causes your muscles to contract, the other picks up varied sensations such as temperature, pressure, pain and the orientation of your joints.

What many people don't realize is that the nerves that supply power to your muscles also supply the energy and nourishment necessary for healing. If you remove a nerve's connection to a muscle, the muscle will die completely. If you remove or restrict a nerve's innervation to a joint, that joint will become arthritic in only a few weeks. These effects are very similar to what would happen if you cut off the blood supply to a tissue. It is imperative to recognize that nerves, beyond giving power to muscles and picking up sensation feedback, also provide nourishment and healing. Too many people, including healthcare professionals, fail to pay attention to this fact.

Relaxed muscles are essential to healthy nerve circulation and proper body function. Full, unhindered circulation allows our nerves to maintain the well-being of the tissues and joints. When we put our tissues through unrelenting wear and tear, even during something as simple as typing without regular breaks or utilizing a work station that is poorly designed, we subject our tendons and muscles to tiny tears that, with time and accumulation, can lead to an overuse injury – even if we had little forewarning before the pain "suddenly appeared." By the time that seemingly sudden pain arrives, your body has already cured itself dozens, even hundreds, of times. The reason the pain won the battle this time is that your body's troops got ambushed.

You see, in spite of its apparent vulnerability to injury, the body routinely uses its nerves and circulation to repair everyday damage.

By the end of the day, especially during rest, it undergoes a net healing: whatever got damaged gets replaced with new tissues so that you'll be okay to get up and go work, play and function again.

However, imagine throwing this process off-balance by decreasing the level of healing because a particular nerve or set of nerves is not able to completely restore itself, or the muscles it supplies, due to constant pressure and poor circulation. When the wear that is inflicted on the body is greater than what it can naturally heal, you leave yourself prone to problems. It is a simple formula: more wear and tear than repair equals injury.

Some of you may have genuine physical symptoms yet report no incidence of injury, repetitive stress disorder or other possible causes of your suffering. Your tests continually show nothing, your symptoms are not in line with your activities, your pain may even move from one spot to another. It is therefore important to touch briefly on another possible culprit, your emotions.

The Emotional Origins of Pain

Once you understand that muscular tension in the neck causes a whole assortment of painful conditions, you can begin to comprehend that not all causes of this tension are strictly physical. The outcome – the suffering – is indeed physical, but the tension that produces the suffering may have a trigger that has little or nothing to do with an actual physical source.

Accepting this idea meets with a great amount of resistance among some people. Many greet this concept with a great deal of skepticism, even anger, at the suggestion that their agony is "all in their head." Let me state again that whatever the source of your muscular tension, whether it's physical or emotional (or a combination of both), your pain is real and absolutely valid. Pain caused from emotional sources is no less horrible, or even different, from the kind suffered with an injury. In some cases it is worse, because injuries typically heal and sufferers can allow themselves to have a positive outlook regarding recovery, while people whose tension stems from emotional causes are often unaware of the true origin of their pain – making their recovery that much more elusive.

Numerous clinical studies have been performed and books written on the subject of pain syndromes caused by deep-seated emotions, and they suggest that suppressed or ignored feelings have a physiological effect on the body's slow-twitch muscles, which include the posterior (rear) muscles of the neck, shoulder, back and buttocks. Once the tension builds in any of these muscles, it is likely to stay and worsen, even without any identifiable cause, and over time this ongoing tension actually alters muscles, tendons and ligaments. The disorder, called Tension Myositis Syndrome (**TMS**), creates an ongoing playground of serious tension and genuine physical suffering that is every bit as excruciating as whiplash, arthritis or any other physical malady.

Think of the last time you saw a really scary movie. Remember how every muscle in your body tensed when the villain suddenly sprang from behind a corner? Now think of the last time you narrowly avoided a collision in your car. The tension you collected *instantly* from that experience probably stayed with you for quite awhile: many minutes, hours or even days. Both examples describe a physical reaction to an emotional source, fear, but in one scenario the reaction passed instantly and in the other it didn't. Since the scary movie was nothing but an imaginary situation, your mind *allowed* your stiffened muscles to expand to their normal state. In the case of the near-miss car accident, however, your brain was fully aware that you came close to catastrophe and it kept your muscles ready to fight or to flee even after the danger passed. The result in such cases is that your muscles remain tight as a drum for a substantially longer period than they should.

This shows how very powerful the mere concept of an unpleasant situation can be on your physical well-being. In syndromes like **TMS**, however, the sufferer typically has no idea that their suppressed emotions are causing them physical problems. If, for example, you leave work every day with a stiff neck, you might easily blame the problem on the fact that you sit in front of a computer all day – a perfectly logical explanation. But your prone posture, of sitting with your hands in front of you for extended periods, may be only part of your problem. And it may not be your problem at all, since some people are unusually unsusceptible to physical injury by luck of their genetics. It could very well be that your X-rays, **MRIs** (magnetic resonance imaging), **CT** (computerized tomography) scans and other tests show no physical evidence of injury because there is none, yet your pain remains extreme and unrelenting. Your stiff neck may not be from typing or commuting (though those activities will certainly worsen your symptoms), but from your anger at your boss for insulting your intelligence or pushing you too hard. Or your frustration may be with a co-worker who isn't pulling his or her weight around the office; it may be sorrow from the loss of a parent; anger at your spouse or one of your children. It may even be caused by your feelings about yourself.

TMS has the same effect on muscles, tendons and ligaments as injury and disease: it causes chronic muscle tension that in turn strains tendons and ligaments, causing *tendonalgia* (tendon and ligament pain), and suppresses circulation to the nerves and muscles, causing aching and stiffness. Because the cause of these reactions is emotional, persons suffering from it are less likely to respond to traditional treatments like medication or even physiotherapy, if the latter is not the variety that encourages relaxation. However, in physiotherapy that does promote relaxation, such as stretching and aerobic activity – both of which are beneficial in relieving emotional anxiety – symptoms do respond favorably. So even if you should determine that **TMS** may be the culprit of your pain, you can treat it with the same methods that I prescribe for my injured or ill patients: the therapies I describe in the "Treatment and Prevention" chapter of this book are designed to relax muscles, whatever the cause of their tension. As an example, let's look at the case of a recent patient of mine:

Maria was sixty-two years old when she came to my clinic with recurrent headaches and neck pain. She also suffered from tension in her upper shoulders and mid-back area. She told me that she'd been diagnosed with high blood pressure, which she managed with medication. Otherwise, tests showed her to be in good health and she reported no injuries that might account for her pain conditions.

During her regular visits to my clinic, Maria often spoke in earnest about the stress of her job, where she had worked for over thirty years. She disliked her job but thought there was no alternative work that would be suitable for her due to her age, lack of education and a slight language barrier because she spoke English as a second language. She also talked of her constant worries about her two adult children's work and personal lives.

Although it seemed apparent that Maria's pain was caused by muscle tension brought on by emotional sources, my treatment of her muscle tension was the same as if she suffered from a physical problem. She responded very well to chiropractic treatment at the clinic, but I knew that would not help her ease her tension over the long-term, so I prescribed regular home treatment with the transcutaneous electrical nerve stimulation (TENS) device I had developed. Initially she reported that Dr. Ho's Muscle Massage System would completely alleviate her symptoms within twenty minutes of application – however on stressful days she continued to experience immediate and severe pain in her neck and shoulders that could bring on a debilitating headache.

Because emotional stress is often ongoing and unpredictable, I recommended that Maria use the TENS system on her neck and shoulders every day, whether she was experiencing stress or not. By stimulating the tense muscles in her neck and shoulders daily, she was able to keep the muscles relaxed. Naturally, on days when she felt especially stressed, her muscles reacted by tensing (which is typical of TMS patients), but her regular TENS therapy prevented the tension from becoming bad enough to create pain. Her daily use of the system was able to prevent the recurrent headache, neck and shoulder pain that she'd been plagued with for years.

Of course even *Dr. Ho's Muscle Massage System* cannot correct the way people *react* to emotional stress – it can only lessen the physical responses to it. What differs between **TMS** sufferers and people dealing with physical maladies is the prevention aspect of treatment. Exercise, stretching and relaxation are good lifestyle habits for anyone to follow and are necessary for all aspects of our health, from prevention to healing. With **TMS**, however, the key to keeping tension at bay is to recognize the sources of your repressed emotions and take logical steps toward confronting your feelings, rather than pushing them from your mind. The end result of this avoidance is muscular tension, and the product is physical misery.

Endocrinologist Dr. Hans Selye is the first doctor credited with drawing attention to how stress affects the body. The emotional stressors can be either external – such as a divorce, a death in the family, work, even illness – or internal, referring to a person's general mindset. Perhaps you have a need to overachieve or be perfect, attempt to be pleasant even when you're miserable, possess a deep inner sorrow, or harbour feelings of self-loathing. Any of these attitudes and others can cause tremendous inner turmoil that often creates muscular tension. Once this tension accumulates enough to cause pain, the body has usually adapted to it as a "normal" state of being and created its own cycle of maintenance. It other words, the pain lingers indefinitely – the reasons why are up for debate. Some doctors and clinicians suggest that the pain serves as an avoidance technique designed to keep you focused on your pain and away from its emotional sources; others believe it is an imperfect but loud "alarm" demanding that you deal with your feelings. In either case, the pain is there and it is all too real, even if your doctor dismisses it because test results reveal no identifiable cause of your agony.

Of course there is no way for this book to identify if you are someone who suffers from **TMS** – that would require some emotional soul-searching on your part and perhaps some type of therapeutic assistance, from a professional or even a trusted friend. But if you suspect that you are someone who "stuffs" your emotions, or if you are under a great amount of personal stress, it is well-worth investigating stress as a possible contributor to your neck tension and any problems associated with it.

If you suffer from chronic pain it is important to note that even if your pain is not from emotional origins, your emotions will influence your recovery. Chronic pain can often produce depression, fear, anxiety, anger, frustration and resentment, and affect your ability to deal with your pain and with those around you. In some people pain can create deep feelings of depression, which can in turn worsen their symptoms. For this reason, all people should view their physical and emotional well-being as equally important parts of the whole.

The Whole Body Approach to Health

Regardless of whether your pain stems from injury, disease or emotional tension, it is imperative to look at your body and mind as harmonious entities. Your physical condition works on your emotional well-being and vice-versa; the two are always interconnected. This connection is reflected in something I call the **Four Pillars of Health:**

1. **The physical pillar** *is your basic anatomy – your skeletal and muscular system. How well is your spine aligned? How well are your joints moving? Are your muscles the appropriate strength and length? This pillar is concerned with minimizing the physical stress on your body.*

2. **The neuro-energetic pillar** *looks after how well your nervous system is flowing, how efficiently your energy travels through your body.*

3. **The chemical pillar** *is the chemical and nutritional aspect. How well are you eating? Do your exercise and sleep patterns support your brain's own chemical balance? How are you eliminating? What types of toxins are you exposed to? All will have an impact on your physical and emotional health.*
4. **The psycho-emotional pillar** *is your spiritual side. How much*

stress are you under? What kinds of emotional trauma do you face now or have you endured in the past? Your attitude toward yourself and your health has a powerful influence on your ability to heal and feel good.

Contemplating all four pillars is what I refer to "looking at the whole body." When I examine patients it is my primary goal to determine what they need – what they can do to help themselves and what I can do as a health professional to assist their recovery. Obviously, the more tools and facts that are at my disposal, the higher the chance that I'll be able to meet a patient's specific needs and provide faster and more complete therapy. The same is true of your healthcare practitioner or team of providers: the more in tune you are with your body and your feelings, the better you'll be able to assist in your own treatment. And further, the better you'll be able to use your understanding during your care at home and during your normal routine.

These four pillars are the foundation of my integrated **Common-Sense** Approach **to your recovery and continued wellness. This approach includes the following:**

1. *Discovering the root cause of your ailment.*
2. *Treatment that zeroes in on the cause(s).*
3. *A routine of specialized, easy exercises.*
4. *Proper rest and correct ergonomics to maximize productivity while reducing fatigue, discomfort and wear and tear on the body.*

Combining clinical treatment with at-home care provides faster and more complete relief than passive involvement, where you rely solely on your healthcare provider to determine the cause and try different "shot in the dark" treatments until you feel better or give up. Equipping yourself with the knowledge to aid in your recovery is one of the most important elements to the success of your care, and reading this book is an important first step.

In the next chapter, we'll tackle the first item listed in the **Common-Sense Approach** to your therapy, discovering the root cause of your disorder. As stated before, if the root cause is an emotional one, you will need to take the appropriate steps toward isolating and dealing with your feelings and how they impact your health. This may include emotional therapy. But since even emotional causes display themselves as physical maladies, and because treatment of your muscle tension is the same in either case, let's take a look at specific pain disorders and diseases in detail to identify how neck muscle tension produces and aggravates them.

Notes:

Identifying the Problem

Most neck pain and dysfunction, as well as the disorders associated with them, are caused by some sort of injury to the soft tissues of the neck, whether it be from trauma, sudden or inappropriate movement, repeated or prolonged activities, or disuse. Even poor posture, such as stooping one's head or cradling the phone for long periods, can cause neck strain. The inflammation or irritation of the neck muscles can in turn cause a laundry list of problems, from migraines to shoulder pain to so-called "tennis elbow."

If you do happen to be afflicted with neck pain, headaches or any other dysfunction or symptoms I describe in this book, once again I strongly urge you go to your doctor for a diagnosis and to receive appropriate testing. It is important to rule out less common but very serious possible causes of neck stiffness and pain, such as the flu, meningitis, even heart disease; or of headaches, such as a rare but serious pathology like aneurysms.

After all, any proper diagnosis relies 95 percent on *listening* and only 5 percent on tests, and clearly only a live person can listen to your symptoms. The intent of this book is to help you avoid what I call "medical mayhem" – the endless bureaucracy of tests, references and prescriptions that address only your symptoms and do not treat your condition. The more you know, the faster and better your chances of real and ongoing pain relief. If you have yet to see your doctor, or if you plan to go in for additional treatment, I encourage you to keep a "diary" of your condition – where you feel pain, what times during the day or night, what things may precede the worsening of your pain and so forth. It will help your doctor to isolate your problem and aid you in your prescribed and at-home treatments.

This chapter will discuss how tension of neck muscles affects the distinct nerves involved with various common maladies. Some, like a stiff neck, are obvious; others, like tenosynovitis of the thumb, may surprise you. As stated previously, the neck is much more important than most people understand. This lack of appreciation causes many associated problems and enables pain to continue much longer than it should. By seeing how it affects the body as a whole, we can move toward recovery.

What Nerves Are Causing My Pain?

Let's take a close look at the crucial nerves that can cause head, neck and shoulder aches when injured, overused, misused or neglected. The spine is composed of thirty-three interlocking bones called vertebrae, twenty-four of which form a flexible column. The remaining nine bones of the sacral and coccygeal sections at the tail of the spine are fused in adults and are called "false vertebrae" since they permit no movement.

Just below the skull are the seven vertebrae of your neck (classified as C1 - C7), forming what is called the *cervical spine*. Just below it we have twelve more vertebrae (T1-T12) that form the *thoracic spine*. The *lumbar spine*, which consists of five vertebrae

(L1-L5), supports your lower back. In between every two vertebrae segments there is an intervertebral disc to provide shock absorption, and a spinal nerve that exits each corresponding vertebra through a hole, or *foramen*, to connect to different regions of the body. Each nerve has a distinct pathway and outline and if there is damage to or a restriction of one of these nerves, pain, numbness or weakness may be felt anywhere along the its route to the head, shoulder, upper arm, elbow, forearm or hand.

The direction and operation of these nerves dictate the proper function, or the painful dysfunction, of these particular areas.

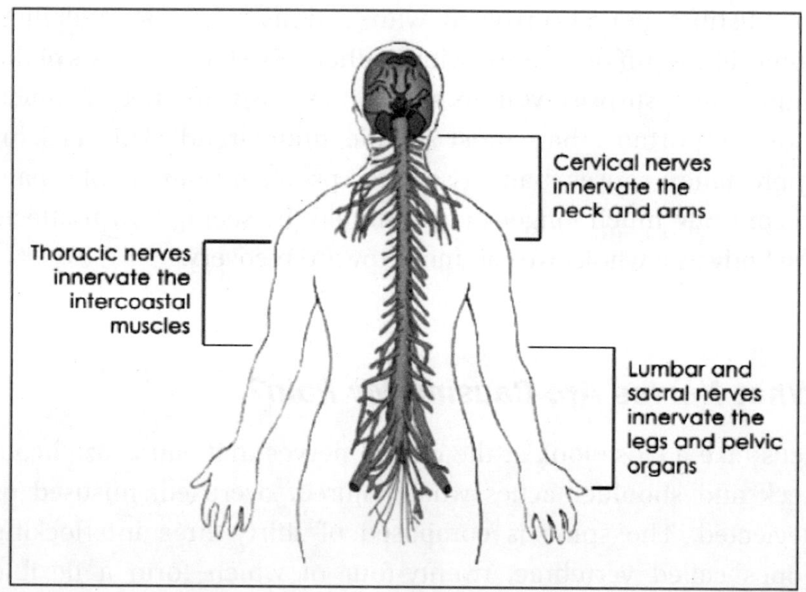

The eight pairs of cervical nerves (C1-C8) are labeled in the same fashion as the vertebrae to pinpoint which vertebra they exit, one from each side to supply the left and right sides of the upper body. There is no eighth cervical vertebra, so the eighth cervical nerve emerges between the seventh vertebra of the neck and the first vertebra of the upper back (T1).

Because they sit just beneath the cervical nerves and also enter the trapezius muscles, the T1 through T6 nerves of the thoracic spine are also relevant to upper body pain conditions. These exit from the spinal cord along the upper back. Each nerve pair supplies feeling and control to specific areas of the head or upper body:

- *C1-C2* — **services the head and neck:** *Located just beneath the base of the skull, any interference with these nerves can cause migraine or tension headaches, fatigue, dizziness, vertigo, insomnia, pressure behind the eyes, an inability to concentrate, sinus pressure and pain, and tenderness in the jaw area (as with temporal mandibular joint — TMJ — disorder).*

- *C3* — **upper/mid-neck:** *Disturbing this nerve pair in the upper/mid-neck area can cause local pain in the upper and middle neck.*

- *C4* — **mid-neck:** *Aggravation of this nerve pair at the mid-neck will cause localized neck pain, stiffness and limited mobility.*

- *C5 - C6* — **lower neck/upper back:** *Suppression of these nerves at the base of the neck will cause lower neck pain, pain in the shoulder joint(s) and weakness in the shoulder muscles. Importantly, the health of these nerves and their circulation has a direct affect on the healing of shoulder bursitis, rotator cuff tendinitis and tennis elbow.*

- *C7* — **upper back:** *When irritated, the nerve that sits where your neck merges with your upper back can cause pain in the lower neck, upper shoulder, wrist and hand and weakness in your elbow, wrist and hand. Its dysfunction can also cause numbness and an achy feeling in the forearm. This is the nerve pair implicated in carpal tunnel syndrome. It is also instrumental in the healing of* *shoulder bursitis, rotator cuff tendinitis, tennis elbow, golfer's elbow and tenosynovitis of the thumb or forefinger.*

- *C8 –* **upper back:** *The impingement of this nerve pair, situated in your upper back, will cause virtually identical symptoms to those described for C7, but in addition can cause pain on the medial side of the elbow, wrist and hand (in line with the pinky finger). It also affects the healing of golfer's elbow.*

- *T1 –* **first nerve pair of the thoracic spine:** *Irritation of the T1 nerve can cause shoulder pain, spot pain beside the shoulder blade and even cause pain in the chest. Compression of the nerves as far down as T6 (the mid-back) can cause referral pain in the upper limbs in a pattern similar to C5-C8.*

The Cervical Nerves – a Closer Look

The very first nerve pair of the spine, located just below the skull at the hairline (C1) is called the *suboccipital*. The suboccipital nerve pair is extremely critical in the diagnosis and treatment of any head-related pain because it links to the nerves around the skull and inside the head. The C2 nerve pair (the *greater auricular*) is about half an inch farther down and also partially exits to the head. If either of these nerves is irritated, it can produce related disorders such as headaches, fatigue, insomnia, dizziness, pressure behind the eyes and/or a band-like throbbing across the forehead.

The remaining spinal nerves join together to form combinations of peripheral nerves called *plexuses*. A plexus is a jungle of nerves that is formed by converged nerve roots from the spine that then branch off to different areas of the body. The nerves of the neck have two *voluntary* plexuses (voluntary means they are dedicated to deliberate movement, like raising your arm or opening your mouth). The first four cervical nerves (C1-C4) form what is called the *cervical plexus,* which engages sensory information for the back of head, the front of the neck and the upper part of the shoulders. Nerve roots from the lower four cervical nerves (C5-C8) and the first thoracic nerve (T1) converge in a pattern called the *brachial plexus,* which is involved in almost all functions (and malfunctions) of the upper limbs.

The brachial plexus begins from the lower five pairs of nerve roots that extend from the C5-T1 vertebrae of the lower neck and upper back, and combines these nerve roots into larger nerve "trunks." They later divide into five major nerves that serve the soft tissues and joints of the shoulders, elbows, wrists and fingers. These major nerves are called the radial, the ulnar, the medial, the axillary and the musculocutaneous nerves. Since these five nerves of the brachial plexus are serviced by nerves that exit the spinal cord from C5-T1, all are directly affected by tension in the muscles of the neck, upper back and shoulders.

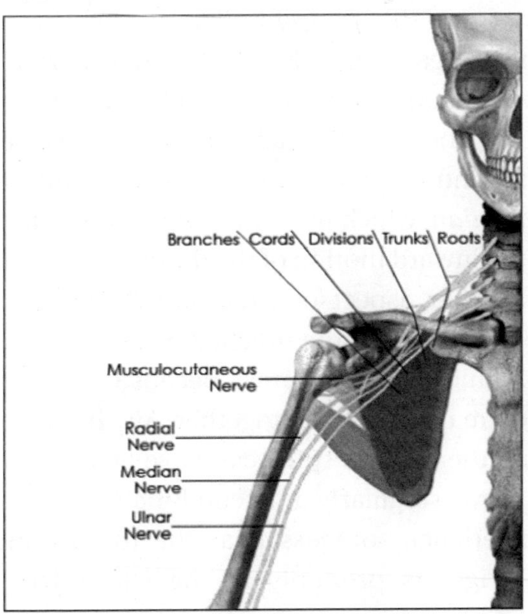

Nerve inflammation in the region from C5 through T1 can cause dysfunction of the extremities – anything from rotator cuff problems to elbow pain to wrist and finger numbness. All these nerves travel from your neck through the brachial plexus to different areas of the upper body, so the most effective and long-term treatment for say, golfer's elbow, usually begins with treating the appropriate nerve site at the neck, rather than by simply treating the site where pain appears.

In practically all the cases I see in my practice, once a patient tells me the location of his or her upper body pain I can form a good idea of where the source is. If they have shoulder pain alone, for example, it is most likely related to a C5 nerve. If they have a problem with "tennis elbow" it is most likely related to C6. The idea that a stiff neck could make your elbow hurt is a strange concept to some people, but it is important to remember that it is the cervical nerves' responsibility to carry information to and from the brain, not to collect it. The cervical nerves collect their information from the *peripheral nerves* of the upper body, including those organized within the brachial plexus. The brachial plexus' nerves include the *axillary,* which innervates the shoulder and upper arm; the *radial,* which innervates the extensors of the elbows, wrists and fingers, as well as the outward motion of the thumb; the *median,* which innervates the middle elbow, wrist and fingers and the inward motion of the thumb; and the *ulnar,* which innervates another aspect of wrist and finger movement. Any irritation to the nerves of the brachial plexus is likely to produce similar and multiple symptoms, because these nerves work together and are often abused together. Any impingement of the nerves exiting the cervical spine can have an effect on any of the nerves they serve, singularly or in combination.

If you experience soreness near the thumb and the index finger, the origin is probably in the C6 and/or C7 nerves.

Insufficient circulation in the C6, C7 and/or the T1 nerves can also cause shoulder pain, since these nerves all enter the *trapezius muscles,* which run from the base of your skull down your neck, across your shoulder and into the upper portion of your back. If you tilt your chin toward your chest, you'll feel the upper part of your trapezius muscle along your neck and upper back stretch. If you shrug your shoulders, you'll feel the muscles of the *levator scapulae,* which run down either side of your neck and to the upper aspect of your shoulder blade.

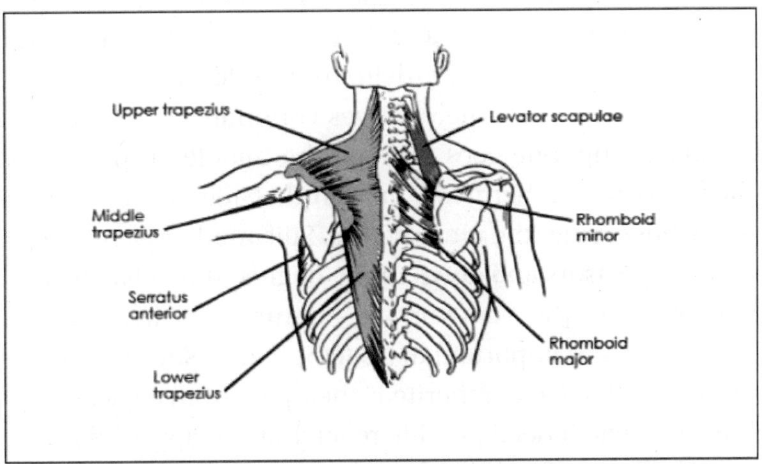

Both the trapezius and the levator scapulae muscles are common tension areas in people. Many patients also experience pain a bit farther down between the shoulder blades, which is the lower end of the trapezius muscle. There, it is affected by the upper thoracic nerves – T1 as far down as T6. A notable characteristic of the trapezius muscle is that it contains a high proportion of "slow-twitch" muscle fibres, enabling extensive and ongoing use. Slow-twitch muscles, which are predominantly those in the posterior (rear) aspect of the body, are especially vulnerable to tension and spasm, and that tension can spread from one slow-twitch muscle to another.

The Spreading Nature of Pain

Sometimes problematic nerves initiate pain in a far-off muscle tissue because inflammation can spread from one muscle to the muscle next to it. Many people experience shoulder blade pain because their tight neck muscles create tension in the adjacent levator scapulae muscles of the upper shoulder. This enables the irritation of nerves at the lower part of the neck to cause upper shoulder pain. Likewise, muscles in the shoulder and upper back can become excruciatingly contracted and, through nerves that run beneath the collarbone and down the arm, inflammation can spread to the front shoulder (deltoid) muscles and to the chest's pectoral muscles. From there nerves continue to move down the arm and split up: one goes through the middle of the wrist (the median nerve); another goes through the side of the wrist along the baby finger side (the ulnar nerve). Still another passes through the elbow extensors and down to the fingers (the radial nerve).

Because of the networking nature of irritation and inflammation, it is important to treat the source site of pain events. Treating sites that have "inherited" their pain from adjacent nerves and muscles will indeed provide relief, but therapy is less likely to be as effective and long-lasting as treating the point of origin, which in upper body maladies is almost always the neck and upper back. Not sure if your shoulder pain is being caused by an impinged C5 or C6 nerve? No problem. One lucky thing about the neck's small size is that you can easily treat whole areas of the cervical spine at once and successfully address your tension-related dysfunction without having to pinpoint the exact spot of origin. Headaches require treatment of the upper neck; neck pain and stiffness without other symptoms indicate treatment of the mid-neck; and pain, numbness or weakness in the extremities suggests treatment be applied to the lower neck/upper back. And with treatment also applied to the point of pain, such as the shoulder or forearm, you're on your way to not only addressing your pain but also to treating your problem.

Having read that promising statement, you're probably ready to jump ahead to the treatment section and begin implementing my techniques of pain reduction and elimination. But before we proceed, let's look at the many varieties of neck dysfunction and injury and the myriad problems they can cause. It is likely one or two will apply to your situation and it will be helpful if you have at least some idea of what caused your pain problem(s) to begin with.

Neck Dysfunction and Associated Pain Disorders

We know that neck dysfunction and its related syndromes are caused by a number of possibilities. Traditional medicine typically associates these disorders within the categories of sudden injury, disc degeneration (often incorrectly) with age and overuse injury with the soft tissues. Migraine headaches, however, are rarely treated by traditional medicine as a consequence of neck dysfunction, which is why the problem is seldom conquered by MDS – they've been able to limit a degree of suffering in some people through medication, but have achieved little beyond that. I directly associate recurring headaches, both migraine and tension, with neck dysfunction, but this topic is large enough that I have given it its own space in the following chapter.

This chapter will highlight some injuries to the soft tissues that commonly bring patients to my pain clinic. I will also give some real-life examples of patient histories so that you can see a distinct pattern in almost all neck pain disorders: there is usually an event or lifestyle tendency that sets the process silently in motion – an accident that has been long-forgotten, a history of misuse or neglect, or both – followed by some type of work or activity that exacerbates neck/upper back muscular tension. Often compounding the problem are habits and postures that promote immobility of the neck, such as infrequent stretching of the area or sleeping on one's belly.

As you read through the pain syndromes it's likely that at least one will seem familiar. If your doctor has diagnosed you with one of these injuries, you will probably learn more about it here than you did during your fifteen minutes in the doctor's office. If you haven't yet had a consultation, you can see which symptoms fit your condition and will be able to assist your doctor in his or her diagnosis.

As you read through the following descriptions, think about your life within the past ten to fifteen years – even further back. Was there an event in your life that I would term an "onset event"; that is, one that could have silently begun you on a path of neck muscle stiffness, disc degeneration and/or compromised mobility? It could have been a common event such as a car accident, or a seemingly minor one involving the head, neck or shoulder, such as a pulled muscle; it could have been a sports injury, or a direct blow to the head, neck or upper back. Typical "onset events" include:

- *Whiplash injuries from an incident such as a car accident.*
- *Working at a computer for extended periods of time.*
- *Waking in the morning with neck spasm.*
- *Working daily with your head down and/or turned to one side.*
- *A direct blow to the neck, head or shoulder.*
- *Activities that keep the neck twisted, such as squeezing the telephone receiver between your neck and shoulder.*
- *Sleeping on your chest with your neck turned to the side.*
- *Sports-related neck and shoulder injuries.*
- *Curvature of the spine from poor posture or scoliosis.*

- *Chronic or sudden emotional overload.*
- *Degeneration of the discs in the neck related to age or abuse.*
- *The onset of disease, such as arthritis.*

Your may recall no specific onset event, but you must also review your physical activity or, just as important, your *inactivity*. As with the elbow-in-the-cast example I used in a previous chapter, your onset event could simply have been years of neglect to the muscles of your neck and/or upper back. Try to be as honest and accurate as possible as you assess your lifestyle. Accidents are usually random events and if you've suffered one or many, it was nothing more than a bit of bad luck; if you've led a largely sedentary life, you have the opportunity to change it for the better; and if you have a chronic condition such as fibromyalgia (which I address fully in chapter 5 or rheumatoid arthritis, these are just conditions that occur among certain people, through no fault of the sufferer. But in all cases, treating and managing your pain is not only possible, but will be much easier and more effective than you've probably been previously led to believe.

Let's begin with the most common conditions that bring people to my pain clinic: repetitive stress disorders, or **RSD**s (also known as repetitive strain or cumulative strain injuries, or cumulative trauma disorders). **RSD**s are overuse (or improper use) injuries that are most often *felt* in the upper extremities, but whose origins are usually neck strain. An **RSD** can strike on one side (usually the dominant side, since a right-handed person, for example, uses the right arm far more than the left), or it can strike both sides at once when jobs or activities require that both arms, wrists or hands be involved on duty.

RSDs can occur to any muscles and soft tissues that are strained repetitively over time. In fact, the neck and shoulder muscles are usually the first that become strained from computer or assembly work, and the muscles frequently ignored by traditional medicine – which is why the associated maladies recur. Left untreated, repetitive stress of the neck and shoulder will contribute to the onset of a long list of disturbing symptoms such as carpal tunnel syndrome, shoulder tendinitis and migraines. Understanding the anatomy of pain and the mechanism of RSDs in the neck and shoulders will enable you to live life without these painful symptoms, so let's quickly review how pain begins.

How Neck and Shoulder Problems Cause Repetitive Stress Disorders

1. Basic neck structure

The seven vertebrae that form the cervical spine are supported by groups of refined muscles. The head requires the neck's posterior muscles to work constantly to keep it balanced and mobile. Delicate nerves exit between the vertebrae and travel through a network of muscles in the neck and down to the shoulders, elbows, wrists and fingers. These spinal nerves have two basic functions: they receive sensation and they supply electrical impulses to the muscles of the neck, shoulders and upper limbs.

2. Course of repetitive strain injury to neck and shoulder

The neck muscles are designed to move in a large range of motion. They are not designed to hold the head in a static position over time, which allows isometric contraction of the muscles. With most computer and assembly work, the long hours of isometric contraction of the neck muscles cause them to become tense and shortened. This begins a cycle of dysfunction.

Remember:

- *Chronically contracted muscles release noxious chemicals that cause local muscle ache, and further tightening that continues even during rest (segmental facilitation).*
- *Tight upper neck muscles irritate and pinch the nerves that run from the upper neck to the head, causing headaches, fatigue, insomnia, dizziness, blurry vision and an inability to concentrate.*
- *Tight lower neck and upper shoulder muscles can aggravate the nerves that run down the upper limbs. Depending on which nerve is being pinched, the symptoms will vary from shoulder, elbow, forearm and/or wrist pain, to pain, numbness and tingling in the hands. Most people who suffer repetitive strain of the muscles of the neck and upper back will eventually suffer from an RSD somewhere in their upper limbs.*

Why are we so prone to these problems? As I've mentioned often in this text, the modern North American lifestyle of overwork and lack of regular movement has led to a huge increase of many common pain conditions, including repetitive stress disorders. The average person works longer days and more days per year than in past generations, has more demands placed on him/her and takes fewer breaks. We also do less exercise to keep taxed muscles and ligaments loose and strong. When I say exercise, allow me to point out that I may not be referring to the first idea that comes to your mind, which is an aerobic activity like jogging or cycling. Certainly they are wonderful examples of exercises to maintain and improve one's health, but the kind that I refer to here is the routine exercise that used to be part of a normal day – walking to the store, for example, or through the park or to the post office, gardening, taking a quick swim on a hot day, dancing around the room with your spouse – small events that take only a few minutes. They may not do for your heart what thirty minutes of jogging would, but they were once part of normal living and they kept our muscles loose and free of waste chemicals, maintained lubrication of our joints, aided flexibility and naturally elevated our sense of well-being. But suburban sprawl has put an end to a lot of the walking we once did – since many people live in neighbourhoods surrounded by nothing but other houses, a trip to the store usually involves getting into a car. The natural neck movements involved in the typical social events enjoyed by past generations has been largely replaced by hours in front of the TV, and many kids now think "playing" exclusively means playing video games. Our jobs keep many of us inactive as we spend long hours at desks or in our cars (the average commuter spends an hour a day going to and from his/her place of employment) and that adds up to a lot of hours of limited movement.

Of course kids can and do suffer from stress disorders as well, most often from playing games or sports that require redundant movements, like pitching a baseball or cycling for long periods, particularly when the activity is performed using bad body mechanics or when it exceeds his or her physical capabilities. Kids are brave and resilient: they take no notice that their arms ache from pitching at an angle that puts too much pressure on their elbows, or that their shoulders burn after a long day of basketball practice. Nor are they likely to care much if their thumbs ache from playing video games for hours on end. Kids have always indulged in this kind of optimism and it's a splendid outlook. But sadly, kids are in worse shape than ever before, so their irregular sports events can create more stress on the body than exercise. Even so, most likely the pain will eventually disappear, but the problem often never completely goes away and becomes a lifelong reminder of their casual neglect.

So we have a foundation of weak and inflexible muscles that come under the stress of repeated or prolonged activities like typing, carrying trays and other objects, weekend tennis or golf, stirring, mixing, writing, turning knobs, pushing keys, lifting, bending, leaning, grabbing, etc. After a while, we may develop aching, gnawing pain that can persist for hours, days or months at a time, or come and go without warning. Some of the most common repetitive stress disorders are those affecting the hands, fingers, forearms, elbows and shoulders and usually involve a particular syndrome. A *syndrome* is a group of symptoms that collectively characterize a particular disease or abnormal condition. Syndromes commonly involve areas of the body where demands are high and space is limited.

RSDs — Pain Syndromes of the Body's Tunnels, Outlets and Cuffs

One thing that the tunnels, outlets and other passageways of our bodies share is that there's a lot going on in a cramped space. Compare these areas to a commuter train crammed to capacity: it takes only one passenger becoming irritated enough to shove someone leaning against him, and suddenly the whole car is hot and filled with tension. These small spaces within our upper bodies have a lot of responsibility, get a lot of use, and house a lot of nerves and tendons inside a tiny area. Further, they are directly affected by neck muscle tension, which is the perfect formula for an overuse injury.

Overuse injuries are caused by excessive or unaccustomed use and are marked by pain and loss of muscle function, weakness, and a loss of control, quickness and accuracy of movement.

Who suffers most from such injuries? Unfortunately, RSDs can happen to almost anyone of any age, but some people are more prone than others. I find that those who suffer most are people who do computer work, since such work requires long hours of sitting, hunching, immobility and forward hand movement like typing and mouse manipulation; people who work in assembly jobs, from factory work to the food service, because they must continually repeat the same lifting, twisting or other movement; and people who play musical instruments, since they typically sit or stand in the same position when they play and must perform specific repeated finger, hand and/or arm movements, often in combination with long periods of bearing weight at an awkward angle (such as holding a guitar with a strap supported near the junction of the neck and shoulder). Among computer workers and musicians in particular, injury is often associated with the increased time and intensity of the activity and an overly tense technique, such as pounding piano or keyboard keys with rigid fingers, or keeping the wrists bent.

These repeated motions, commonly coupled with long periods of little head and neck movement, can set people up for any number of pain syndromes.

Let's look at the most common:

Carpal Tunnel Syndrome

Musicians, computer users, food service workers, graphic designers, athletes, manual labourers and others who require repeated, rapid or twisting motions of their hands and/or wrists can develop a sometimes agonizing pain condition called *carpal tunnel syndrome*. Even everyday events like cooking can cause CTS if it requires you to use your hands and wrists to commit the same motion over time, as you might by stirring food.

Like almost all repetitive stress disorders of the upper body, CTS begins in your lower neck and upper back, where nerves collect to form the brachial plexus, which runs down through the anterior triangle of the neck, through the collarbone, through the shoulder and then branches off down to your arms in different distributions. One of these branches from the brachial plexus is the *median nerve*, and it passes through the carpal tunnel, the small bony passageway at the base of your palm where it meets your wrist, to your hand to enable sensation in some of your fingers and your thumb. If you extend your arm with the palm up and make a fist, you'll notice two tendons that look like parallel wires near your wrist – this is where the median nerve passes into your hand.

If a cervical nerve is irritated at the base of the neck or upper back, inflammation and swelling can spread to the median nerve, making it very difficult for it to go through the carpal tunnel. Because the carpal tunnel is a very snug space to begin with, any swelling – no matter how slight – can cause pressure on the median nerve and make the simplest movements of the hands and fingers difficult. When irritated, the median nerve is extremely sensitive and even a minuscule amount of pressure will cause it to become symptomatic. Symptoms can include soreness or a weird tingling sensation all the way down the arm, weakness, clumsiness and a lack of sensation in the fingers. In severe cases, you can get a concert of misery including shoulder, elbow, wrist and finger pain and weakness, causing the sufferer horrible discomfort doing even the most rudimentary of tasks.

The carpal tunnel is open widest when the wrist is in line with the hand, so pressure on the median nerve can be relaxed by simply straightening the wrist. Most people report that their symptoms are lessened or even disappear when their arms are at their sides – when the wrist is fully extended and the tunnel is wide enough to permit even swollen nerves to circulate. For this reason, splints are often provided to people suffering **CTS**, so their wrists will stay straight during sleep and while performing tasks like typing or assembling. To keep the median nerve from rubbing against the walls of the carpal tunnel, it is important to practice tasks involving the wrist with a "floating" hand posture: in other words, type, assemble and work with your wrists in a straight line, not curved upward or downward.

Interestingly, the median nerve does not supply all your fingers, but only the first and second, the thumb and part of the middle finger. The remainder are innervated by another nerve, the *ulnar*. But because both nerves are affected by muscle tension in the same area of the neck and upper back, frequently both these nerves are irritated and produce symptoms simultaneously. Symptoms can become bad enough that sufferers must wake up during the night so they can shake their hands to get rid of the tingling sensations. If the irritated median nerve is left untreated for a long time, it can lead to atrophy of the muscles it serves, resulting in an inability to pinch and even in permanent muscle damage.

Carpal tunnel syndrome is most commonly attributed to an excess of a particular motion involving the wrist or hands that eventually causes inflammation. In many cases, however, the inflammation may disappear and the pain stays. This is more accurately attributed to *tendinosis* (see following section). Other causes can include rheumatoid arthritis, being overweight, diabetes, thyroid disease and even pregnancy. Less commonly, **CTS** can be caused by a fracture in the wrist and/or hand, which can bring about swelling and sometimes even change the shape of the tunnel as the bones heal. I've seen cases of **CTS** so severe that the sufferer actually undergoes surgery to widen the carpal tunnel, but in my experience this treatment is seldom useful. Widening the tunnel does not treat the irritated median nerve, and the patients still complain of symptoms afterward. I liken it to ripping out the frame of a doorway to make room for a door that's become swollen from summer heat. It is bad medicine to alter a healthy area of the body to compensate for an ailing one, especially when proper treatment has not been applied to cure the malfunction at its common source: the neck. The cervical nerve C7, which extends to the median nerve, is where effective treatment should begin.

How can this condition be treated successfully? Let's take a look at a real-world example:

> *Cynthia is a thirty-six-year-old woman who came to my clinic with numbness, pain and a loss of strength in both hands. She reported dropping glasses and other objects, indicating trouble with the motor coordination of the fingers. She stated that her hand pain had started gradually about two years before and had since continued to get worse. She would get up most mornings with severe numbness in both hands and sometimes the pain would wake her up in the middle of the night. Cynthia was a stay-home mom and looked after her two children full-time. She could not recall any injuries to her hand or wrist and pointed out no regular activities that might cause strain.*
>
> *Prior to visiting my office, she saw her family doctor who diagnosed her as having carpal tunnel syndrome. She was prescribed pain and anti-inflammatory medications that provided her inadequate relief. As her condition worsened, her doctor referred her to physiotherapy for ultrasound and exercise therapy. She was custom-fitted with a pair of wrist splints that she wore during sleep. Her condition did not improve significantly after eight weeks of physiotherapy, so she stopped going for treatments.*
>
> *Her history revealed that she was in good health, but she did report that she'd been involved in a minor car accident about five years prior, when the car she was driving was hit from*

behind while she was stopped at a traffic light. She didn't sustain any major injuries but recalled having a sore neck and some headaches for several weeks afterward. These minor symptoms were relieved by over-the-counter pain medication and, because her symptoms were slight, she sought no medical help.

My examination of her neck revealed significant restriction in movement. Her range of motion was approximately fifty percent of normal. The muscles of the back, sides and lower part of her neck and the muscles of her upper shoulders were hardened and tender when touched. When I applied pressure on the neck at certain "tender points" at the sides, she reported an uncomfortable sensation in both arms. When pressure was maintained on these points for about thirty seconds, she noted the numbness and pain in her hands became more intense. This indicated that the nerves from her neck to her arms were highly irritated and that any slight addition of pressure aggravated them instantly. Interestingly, examination of her wrist showed no signs of dysfunction, suggesting the actual site of her agony was functioning properly.

Cynthia was advised to use a transcutaneous electrical nerve stimulation (TENS) device at the site of her wrist pain, as well as on her neck and shoulders to increase circulation and rid those muscles of built-up noxious chemicals. She treated herself at home four to five times every day, for about thirty minutes each time. After only one treatment she stated that she experienced immediate relief; after the first week she reported that she no longer awakened in the morning with pain or numbness in either hand. By the second week, she reported that her episodes of clumsiness had ceased completely.

After about four weeks of daily home treatment with my specially designed TENS therapy device, Dr. Ho's Muscle Massage System, she felt that she had made a full recovery and thereafter used the device only as needed. The electrical stimulus relaxed her neck and shoulder muscles while stimulating conduction to the nerves that run through her neck to her wrist. As part of her home treatment program, Cynthia followed the motion and strength restoration exercises recommended in the "Treatment and Prevention" chapter..

Cynthia is happy with her recovery – she now sleeps deeply and without pain, and wakes up refreshed and energetic.

What this example demonstrates is that the *cause* of Cynthia's disorder was initially misdiagnosed and improperly treated by her doctor. Her condition likely would have remained, because her wrist had been blamed for her problem when in reality it started in her neck and shoulders.

Cubital Tunnel Syndrome

Cubital tunnel syndrome is caused by a compression of the ulnar nerve, which passes through the *cubital tunnel* at the inside of the elbow on its way toward the hand. This tunnel, at the bone on the inside of your elbow (the funny bone), is supported by a network of ligaments and muscles that, when injured or inflamed, can create pressure on the ulnar nerve. Repeated flexion and extension of your elbow, or the resting of your forearm on a hard surface (like a desk or armrest) or against a sharp edge, can cause the ulnar nerve to become irritated or pinched. This disorder can result in pain, numbing and/or tingling of the fourth and fifth, or ring and pinky fingers, which the ulnar nerve services. It can also cause hand pain and clumsiness, which sometimes causes it to be mistaken for carpal tunnel syndrome. People with arthritis and diabetes are at higher risk of coming down with this condition, as are those who spend a lot of time leaning on their elbows.

Jobs associated with this disorder are those that require constant use of a telephone handset, the playing of musical instruments, assembly-line work, sign language, machine operation and long-distance driving. As with carpal tunnel, the key to recovery is to treat the tension in the lower neck/upper back muscles, reduce stress to the elbow(s), get rid of inflammation and increase circulation to promote healing and prevent reinjury. The C8 and T1 nerves are the usual sites in the neck that can cause or aggravate this syndrome.

Radial Tunnel Syndrome

This injury, like carpal and cubital tunnel syndromes, results from compression of a nerve. In this case it is the *radial nerve,* which travels along the outside of the elbow and is irritated by prolonged wrist and/or finger flexion, forceful pushing or pulling actions, regular bending of the wrist and constant gripping and twisting. Although the cause is different, the symptoms of RTS are similar to and often mistaken for *lateral epicondylitis,* or "tennis elbow," since pain is felt in the same spot just outside the elbow and gets worse with continued use of the affected arm. In tennis elbow, however, the pain is typically felt directly where the tendon attaches to the *lateral epicondyle,* the outer bone of your elbow that sits in line with your shoulder. In radial tunnel syndrome, though, the tender spot is about two inches farther down the forearm, where the radial nerve passes into the large muscle called the *supinator* that runs atop the arm. Irritation of the radial nerve causes it to become constricted within the small tunnel of surrounding muscles and bone at the outer aspect of the elbow.

Common irritants are constant or improper mouse and/or keyboard work, graphic design work, assembly-line tasks, the playing of musical instruments, painting, writing, woodworking and other work requiring one or both arms to be held in front of the body for long periods.

The diagnosis of radial tunnel syndrome can be difficult since it is often mistaken for tennis elbow or even carpal tunnel syndrome. Often the only way a correct diagnosis can be made is with a physical examination that pinpoints the area exhibiting the greatest amount of tenderness. But you'll probably be glad to learn that it isn't imperative for you to know if you suffer from tennis elbow or radial tunnel syndrome in order to treat the source of your pain. Because all three tunnels I describe in this section involve a major nerve – median, ulnar or radial – that receives information from the cervical spinal cord, treating the source of their compression in tight muscles of the lower neck (C5-T1) can relieve all of these syndromes, no matter which nerve is the actual culprit. Isn't that a relief!

Lateral Epicondylitis (Tennis Elbow)

Lateral epicondylitis, or "tennis elbow," is generally considered to be an overuse tendinitis that afflicts the tendon that attaches to the "outer bump" (the *lateral epicondyle*) of the elbow, and causes pain there as well as in the *extensor carpi radialis brevis,* the forearm muscle that enables you to bend your wrist back. If you hold out your arm with your palm facing the floor, this muscle – we'll call it the *extensor muscle* for brevity's sake – will be angled toward the ceiling.

Tennis elbow gets its nickname from the many injuries that result from overuse of the extensor muscles and tendons that tennis players use to hit a backhand shot. Of course, this is but one cause of the condition and you certainly don't have to play tennis to suffer from it. Ironically you can also get it from playing golf (and you can get golfer's elbow from playing tennis), as well as from myriad other things such as using power tools or juggling (yes, juggling!). Any repetitive movement that tears or irritates the extensor muscles and tendon attachments of the forearm (the soft tissues that enable the wrist to bend backward and your forearm to twist your wrist) can cause the disorder. Frequent backward motion of the wrist (extension), turning the hand palm-side up, or lifting an object with the elbow held straight are common activities that aggravate these tissues.

The severity of the pain and damage can get to the point where you may have great difficulty twisting doorknobs, washing dishes, typing, using tools or playing sports. It can make any activity difficult, especially performing your job. Take, for example, a recent patient named David:

> *David is a forty-two-year-old gentleman who came to my clinic with agonizing pain in the outer corner of the elbow that radiated down his forearm. The elbow pain was made worse whenever he made a gripping action with his hand. David reported that the pain started suddenly about two years before and had gotten progressively worse. At the time of his visit, he said that he was unable to do his job as a painter because of his elbow pain.*
>
> *Previous treatment included anti-inflammatory and pain medications, but they'd provided only temporary relief. He'd*

had two cortisone injections at his elbow, which seemed to help at first but the pain would come back roughly four weeks after each shot. He also had physiotherapy and acupuncture treatments, which did not help significantly.

During the examination I discovered an extremely tender spot over the lateral (outward) side of the elbow. David's forearm muscles were tight and ropey. When I asked him to hold a tight fist and extend his wrist, it elicited severe pain at the elbow. His forearm muscles were quite weak and he was unable to resist any challenge to his wrist extension.

David's medical history revealed a healthy male with no other known health problems. He did mention that whenever he painted, his neck and shoulders would get tight and sore, but that after twenty years on the job he'd more or less accepted the achy feeling as being par for the course.

An X-ray of his elbow showed nothing significant. An X-ray of his neck, however, showed severe degeneration of the joints and cervical discs.

Physical examination of David's neck revealed that his range of motion was approximately 65 percent of normal. His entire neck and upper shoulder muscles were extremely tight and tender, particularly along the sides.

When an upper limb problem persists and continues to get worse even with rest and treatment, it usually indicates that the nerves from the neck aren't fully conducting to the arm. Since David was disabled from work due to the chronic elbow pain, a referral to a neurologist was recommended to initiate a nerve conduction exam. The examination showed a minor loss of nerve conduction in his forearm.

I prescribed a treatment for David that included a regular home care program using Dr. Ho's Muscle Massage (TENS) system. He applied the electrotherapy device daily to his elbow at the site of pain, as well as the muscles in his forearm, neck and upper shoulder, for eight weeks. He treated himself five to six times per day, at least twenty to thirty minutes each time. He also refrained from certain activities that could aggravate the problem, like gripping with his hand and twisting or extending his wrist. He also wore an elbow support to remind him to treat his elbow gently. He regularly did a very light stretching exercise to lengthen the forearm muscles and take pressure off the tendon attachment at the elbow. He also rotated his head from side to side every thirty minutes to help restore movement in his neck.

After one week of home treatment, he noticed a significant improvement in his neck movement but his elbow pain remained about the same. After three weeks of daily home treatment, the pain in his elbow began to abate and he was able to grab light objects without discomfort. By the sixth week, he felt that he could return to work as a painter part-time, and by the end of the eighth week, when the strength in his forearm was restored, he returned to work full-time. However, he reported that he still felt some neck tension and stiffness at the end of his workday. Since degeneration of the discs and joints in his neck was already present, I recommended that he use the TENS device at least twice a day – once in the morning and again before bedtime – to keep his muscles relaxed and the nerves conducting. I also instructed him to continue with his neck and elbow exercises so that the pain would stay gone for good. David's commitment to his own care has made the difference and has allowed him to enjoy a remarkable recovery.

Examples like David's are common in my practice, but you may suffer from lateral epicondylitis and have no idea how you got it. Interestingly, although tennis elbow is generally considered to be a type of overuse tendinitis, a great number of people who suffer from it have no history of overusing their arms: no endless sets of tennis or long days working construction. What, then, causes these people to acquire this disorder? In tennis elbow it is usually irritated C7 nerves in the lower neck/upper back that cause the problem, though C8 and T1 may also contribute if they are obstructed as well.

Medial Epicondylitis (Golfer's Elbow)

Medial epicondylitis, or "golfer's elbow," produces the same pain and symptoms as tennis elbow, but on the medial (inside) aspect of the elbow where the bone is tiny and rounded. If you hold your arm with your palm facing skyward, the forearm muscles you see are the forearm flexors, which attach to the inside of the elbow (the *medial epicondyle*). If these flexor muscles are overused they can pull excessively on the attached tendon, causing minute tears and inflammation. Like tennis elbow, golfer's elbow can restrict your ability to grab and hold things because the affected tendon and flexor muscles control your faculty to flex your forearm and make a fist. Treatment of golfer's elbow is usually a bit different from treating tennis elbow, since it typically involves nerves a bit farther down the upper back – the C8 and T1 nerves.

Rotator Cuff Injury

The rotator cuff is a collection of four tendons connecting the bone of the upper arm with the shoulder blade. The rotator cuff's function is to raise, lower and rotate the arm. Aggravation of the tendons within the rotator cuff is a very common problem for the same reason that carpal tunnel syndrome is – a lot of nerves travelling through a cramped space – and it can cause nagging, persistent pain. If the pain is from an overuse injury, like regular lifting at your job, or from a direct blow, it is most likely a soft tissue affliction, such as tendinitis or bursitis, which is why a rotator cuff injury is also called *rotator cuff tendinitis*. However, rotator cuff injuries frequently happen for no apparent reason at all – you just wake up with it one day or notice shoulder pain while performing a normal activity. Age, injury and simple wear and tear can lead to the weakening of the rotator cuff tendons through a condition called impingement, and can result in weakness and pain in the shoulder. In more serious cases of rotator cuff injury or irritation, sufferers can experience "frozen shoulder," a condition that makes it all but impossible to lift objects or elevate the arm beyond shoulder height.

Some medical studies have suggested that part of the reason the rotator cuff is susceptible to injury even with normal use is that the area is one which receives an inadequate blood supply, limiting its ability to fend off normal wear and tear the way most other parts of the body do. Because our shoulders are an integral part of so many activities, the rotator cuff gets more than its share of use and abuse, which may explain why its injury becomes more common as people get older.

Because an ageing or weakened rotator cuff is so vulnerable to injury, it is important that one employ restraint when using the shoulders for any extreme activity, especially lifting heavy objects with arms extended or trying to catch a heavy falling object. Such events can lead to an actual tearing of the rotator cuff, an agonizing condition that often results in the inability to raise one's arm until the tear is treated – either by therapy or, in more serious cases, surgery.

After an initial period of rest and appropriate anti-inflammatory treatment (the vast majority of the time ice will work better than medication in reducing inflammation), the best treatment for most rotator cuff injuries is physiotherapy to restore motion and strengthen the area, lessening the chance of further damage. The best way to continue to avoid ongoing or recurring pain, however, is to increase circulation to the tendons of the shoulder. Because the area is naturally impinged, I find the best way to get blood to the rotator cuff is through electrical stimulation using a **TENS** device such as *Dr. Ho's Muscle Massage System*, not only to the shoulder itself, but in the trapezius muscles of the posterior neck and the levator scapulae muscles where your upper shoulder meets your neck. You'll recall that the brachial plexus contains nerves that innervate the shoulders – more specifically, it serves the axillary nerves that give the shoulder muscles the power to extend your arms over your head, in front of your chest and behind your back. Tension in your lower neck and upper back muscles has a direct effect on your shoulder's ability to function and heal properly. In most cases of rotator cuff pain that I treat, tension in the muscles supplied by the C5 and C6 nerves is the primary source of pain and weakness felt in the shoulder(s). The C7 nerve plays its part, too, since it affects the healing of rotator cuff and shoulder tendinitis, as well as shoulder bursitis. If the nerves from the neck suffer any kind of limited conduction on their service path to the shoulder, they can cause ongoing problems within the rotator cuff – which is by its nature starved for circulation – and symptoms can become so serious that simply raising your arm or lifting anything, even something light, becomes excruciating.

Treatment at the rotator cuff disorder's origin, the C5-T1 nerves, usually provides greater and more long-term relief than treating only the site of pain at the shoulder.

Tenosynovitis of the thumb (De Quervain's Syndrome)

The term *tenosynovitis*, which is perhaps harder to say than to explain, means an inflammation of the outer covering, or sheath, of a tendon. This swelling irritates the tendon inside and restricts its movement, and can cause the tendon's surface to become irritated and rough. The thumb has two important tendons, the abductor and the extensor, which control its movement functions. These two tendons share a common sheath, so when the sheath is swollen it affects both tendons and can cause pain, stiffness and weakness not only in the thumbs but in the wrists as well, prompting some health professionals to mistake it for carpal tunnel syndrome. Like CTS, tenosynovitis is typically an overuse injury, but it is caused by different actions – usually those involving forced grasping or frequent gripping motions like filing papers or books, playing certain musical instruments, doing computer work, performing massage, sawing, hammering, screwing and carrying out other carpentry-like activities. Unfortunately, the usual course of traditional medical treatment for carpal tunnel will not relieve the symptoms of tenosynovitis. For example, let's look at another case involving one of my patients:

> *Brenda is a forty-six-year-old graphic designer who visited my office with wrist soreness on the thumb side. Any movement of*

her thumb elicited excruciating shooting pain along the tendon of her thumb at the wrist area. The problem started about a year ago got progressively worse over time. At the time of her visit, she was experiencing pain whenever she did design work at her computer. Previous treatment included anti-inflammatory and pain medication. She also had extensive physiotherapy care for her wrist, including ultrasound, ice and mobility exercises, but it didn't significantly improve her condition. At night she wore a wrist support to prevent movements that could aggravate her condition during sleep. She also consulted with an orthopedic surgeon who recommended wrist surgery to release the pressure inside the tendon sleeve. The surgeon could not affirm that she would be free from pain after the surgery.

Brenda's history showed that working on her computer aggravated her wrist pain. She also noted that her neck often felt stiff and achy in the morning and that she often felt tired when she awoke, even with adequate sleep. Her general health was good but she did complain of experiencing migraine headaches about once a week.

An X-ray of her wrist provided no explanations.

Upon my examination, there were a few signs that clearly showed that Brenda's neck was not functioning properly. I discovered that her neck muscles were very tight and tender and that her range of motion was only about 60 percent of normal. When I applied pressure to her neck muscles, I discovered that she had severe tenderness all along her neck, including both sides. Pressure to the lower right side of her neck caused her to have an aching sensation that travelled down her arm into her hand.

I recommended that she use Dr. Ho's Muscle Massage (TENS) system at home on the tendons of her thumb and the muscles that move the thumb. I also showed her where to apply the pads on her neck to treat the C7 nerve roots. The electrotherapy stimulation relieved the pain and inflammation within the tendon sheath, relaxed the muscles attached to the tendon, and decreased the tensile stretch on the tendon. Most importantly, the device relaxed the muscles in the neck and removed pressure from the nerves that run from the neck to the hand, and promoted blood circulation and nerve conduction from the neck to the hand to encourage faster natural healing.

Her home treatment included application to her wrist, forearm and neck three times per day, at least twenty minutes each time. As part of her rehabilitation, she mobilized her wrist and thumb joint by gently moving it within her comfort range several times a day. To restore normal neck motion, she mobilized her neck by turning her head from side to side within her comfort range ten times every thirty minutes.

Brenda noticed a significant improvement the first day she started to treat herself and enjoyed a very deep sleep without interruption on account of her wrist pain. After four weeks, she was able to work at her computer without pain, provided she remembered to do her mobilization exercises. She continued with the home treatment plan for another eight weeks and reported that she had regained full movement of her thumb and wrist. Her neck was also greatly improved, though she still required treatment after a night's sleep and again at the end of the day after spending many hours on her computer. Incidentally, she reported feeling much more energetic and had a complete recovery from her migraines. Overall, she was extremely happy with the results.

As I stated before, *traditional* medical treatment for carpal tunnel syndrome will usually provide inadequate relief for thumb tenosynovitis. However, treatment of the C7 nerves at the lower neck/upper back can provide relief for both syndromes. This is wonderful news for those who suffer both maladies concurrently.

Tenosynovitis of the Finger (Trigger Finger)

If you were a gunslinger in the Old West, the cause of "trigger finger" would be obvious and treatment would involve your refraining from frequent shootouts with treacherous hombres. In the modern world, however, tenosynovitis of the finger is a disorder that causes the tendon that supports your first finger to "lock" and create jerky movements when the forefinger is used.

Causes are any that require the first finger to constantly contract, as with shooting: the constant use of spray bottles, grasping handles or hard objects, playing video games or certain musical instruments and operating certain tools. It is less common than tenosynovitis of the thumb (but probably more fun to say you have, since it invites some interesting discussion). Treatment for both disorders converges on the C7 nerves exiting the lower neck/upper back.

Thoracic Outlet Syndrome

Thoracic outlet syndrome results from a compression of nerves and blood vessels comprising the *brachial plexus,* the complex network of motor and sensory nerves that exit the base of the neck near the clavicle (collarbone) and extend to the first and second ribs near the *axilla*, or arm pit. This network provides control, strength and feeling to the arms, hands and shoulder girdle. Pressure on the nerves of the brachial plexus by muscular tension between the cervical spine and the top of the thoracic spine of the upper back (C8 and T1) can cause limited nerve function and suppressed circulation to the arms, hands and shoulders, as well as regions of the head and neck.

Pressure to this nerve system can often be attributed to extensive overhead activities, like painting, woodworking and cleaning, or activities requiring forward reaching such as typing, cashiering, doing assembly work, playing musical instruments, painting, driving, or carrying heavy loads over your shoulder or with your arms extended.

Symptoms of thoracic outlet syndrome include pain and weakness of the upper extremities, clumsiness and/or coldness of the hands, and tiredness, heaviness and limited use of the arms when elevated. The syndrome can also cause extreme stiffness and pain in the neck and shoulders and, because of the brachial plexus' containment of the *subclavian artery and vein*, can cause headaches and numbness or other strange feelings in the face and ear. Very commonly **TOS** is accompanied by a pain in the chest wall, where the brachial plexus passes on its way through the armpit. Other common symptoms include weakness, a pins-and-needles sensation, and pain in the upper extremity. The exact location of the symptoms is dependent upon which nerve is irritated.

A correct diagnosis usually involves your healthcare provider's use of a thoracic outlet syndrome test called the *Selmonosky Triad*. The test involves elevating your hands to check for strength and being examined for swelling, sweating, clumsiness, limited power and movement and strength, tenderness around your collarbone and weakness in your ring and pinky fingers.

Some people have a predisposition for thoracic outlet syndrome and find that even a few months of repetitive work with their upper extremities will produce symptoms. On the other hand, some people show a lesser tendency for the disorder and may require years of repetitive work before any symptoms appear, or their symptoms may be so incidental that they get ignored for a long time. In almost all sufferers, however, the tingling, weakness or heaviness of their arms and hands eventually make it difficult or impossible to perform repetitive work or even everyday functions.

People with thoracic outlet syndrome may have few or many symptoms. Some symptoms, like anterior chest pain, can make diagnosis difficult for doctors unaware of the disorder's roster of indicators.

As you can see, any of these repetitive stress disorders can be anything from a nuisance to a debilitating event. Almost all have root causes in tension of lower neck and upper back muscles. Luckily, all respond well in my experience to treatment that focuses on relieving irritation and stiffness of those muscles. Another thing that RSDs have in common is that they are typically assigned to the categories of injuries known as *tendinitis, tendinosis* and *bursitis.*

What are Tendinitis, Tendinosis and Bursitis?

Simply, these conditions describe different types of injury to the soft tissues. "Soft tissue" refers to the tendons, muscles, bursae and ligaments of our bodies that work in tandem to support a joint and give it function. What are the differences between tendinitis, tendinosis and bursitis? That's a question easier asked than answered because their causes and symptoms are so similar they're almost interchangeable. The only appreciable differences are inflammation (which may or may not be visible to the naked eye) and the precise site of injury, and you certainly can't be expected to be able to identify either. In fact, your doctor may not be able to guess any more accurately than you can. He or she may tell you that you have bursitis without truly knowing, as is commonly the case with shoulder and wrist conditions. Even after tests your doctor may not have a definitive idea: you could show minor inflammation in any of your soft tissues, or several in combination, or you may have no inflammation at all. Typically your doctor will pick one just to give you a diagnosis, then your specialist will pick another, leaving you more confused than ever. The good news? It doesn't much matter whether your sore shoulder or aching wrist is tendinitis, tendinosis or bursitis, because the treatment is materially the same for all three: rest, exercise and stretching. The bad news, of course, is that all three can cause a lot of pain. Let's look at them in turn.

Tendinitis: Tendons are the tough, ropey fibres that attach muscle to bone. The very common pain condition known as tendinitis is an inflammation of those tendons and of smaller tendon-muscle attachments, usually caused by injury or overuse. An inflamed tendon can cause mild to serious pain, diminished strength and limited movement. It can happen suddenly, from landing on the palm of your hand in a fall, for example, which will stress the tendon along your wrist and create swelling. Or it can happen slowly, and begin as an annoyance that turns into pain that is so severe it's actually debilitating, as with carpal tunnel syndrome. Overuse or repetitive movements of a tendon can result in nagging pain, burning, redness, heat, tenderness, joint stiffness and/or limited motion of the affected area or in a related area. Carpal tunnel syndrome, for example, can cause pain not only in the wrist itself, but in the fingers, hand, and all the way up the forearm.

Treatment of tendinitis usually focuses on decreasing inflammation so that physiotherapy or exercise is possible to preserve motion and create strength in the weakened areas. Temporary use of non-steroidal anti-inflammatory drugs (**NSAIDs**) like Aspirin, ibuprofen (Advil) and naproxen sodium (Aleve) can help to reduce inflammation, but should be abandoned once inflammation is gone or if they are allowing you to continue to use, rather than to rest, the affected area. Sometimes the area is restricted so that movement will be minimal until the inflammation diminishes. You've certainly seen people wearing Velcro-strapped splints on their hands and forearms – maybe you've had to wear one yourself. They can help to relieve inflammation, but once the inflammation is gone they should be put on only as needed, and exercises should be implemented to restore movement. Cold therapies such as ice packs are often more helpful in reducing swelling and relieving pain than heat, which can aggravate inflammation.

Interestingly, however, current research on the topic of tendinitis suggests that most people diagnosed with tendon injury have no traceable signs of inflammation, suggesting that most cases of tendinitis might be more correctly identified as *tendinosis.*

Tendinosis: Instead of inflammation of the tendons, tendinosis is caused by a degeneration of the collagen within the tendon's tissues. Because collagen is responsible for giving tendons their strength, its loss can cause afflicted tendons to be susceptible to tiny tears that continue to weaken them and invite further injury or reinjury and subsequent scar tissue. Tendinosis is not only more common than tendinitis, it is somewhat more serious, because it often follows tendinitis as proof of ongoing tendon degeneration and scar tissue buildup. Left untreated, it can sometimes lead to the development of calcium crystals within the tendon, a malady called *calcific tendinitis*, which can cause chronic pain. Therefore, if you are diagnosed with tendinitis it is important to isolate what caused it and to instigate treatment to cure it before it turns into tendinosis.

In all cases, increasing circulation to the affected areas is key, as it facilitates healing and removes waste products from the adjacent muscles. Once pain has been reduced or eliminated, exercises devoted to increasing strength and flexibility are key in helping to prevent its recurrence.

Bursitis: This common problem falls under the same family, but it is caused when a *bursa*, a small sac of fluid that helps the muscles slide easily over other muscles and bones, is overused. Injury or overuse of a joint or tendon can irritate and inflame the bursae, creating a condition known as bursitis. Bursitis often develops quickly, over just a few days, sometimes after a specific injury such as a direct blow (traumatic bursitis), or sometimes after a period of overuse. Usually it will subside in a few days or weeks, provided one avoids the activity that caused it in the first place.

Bursitis can occur at several different places in the body at the same time or be localized to one area. Regular warm-ups and stretching may help prevent bursitis, so do them before activities that require repeated movement or strenuous work. Chances are strong that the problem will recur if steps are not taken to heal, strengthen and stretch the muscles in the areas that first displayed symptoms. It's important not to mask the pain with medication if doing so will cause you to continue to overuse the affected area(s). Sure, a few Advil will enable you to pitch at your company's softball game in spite of your sore shoulder, but at what cost? In the initial stages of tendinitis or bursitis, pain must be viewed as a good thing – it's warning you to pay attention to what you're doing and giving you a constant reminder to knock it off, change how you do it or, at very least, take frequent breaks to allow healing. However, once pain becomes ongoing it is everything from a nuisance to a burden to a curse.

Tendinitis, tendinosis and bursitis can afflict both children and adults, especially those whose jobs or leisure activities require them to perform repetitive tasks, from a desk or labour job to housework, from golf to baseball, even cooking and gardening.

Unless the injured area is allowed to have proper rest and heal fully, these conditions usually get worse. Treatment includes applying ice, doing gentle exercises and stretching to prevent stiffness and increase circulation. Medication can temporarily mask the pain, but this may counterproductively prevent the damaged tendon or bursa to get the rest it needs.

Shoulder Pain

The second most common problem I encounter in patients is tense, achy and sore muscles in the lower neck and upper shoulder area, particularly the trapezius muscle of the posterior neck, shoulder and upper back, and the levator scapulae muscles at the junction of the neck and upper shoulder. The muscles of the levator scapulae (which is Latin for "raiser of shoulder blades," describing its function) attaches above to the cervical vertebrae and below to the upper inside corner (toward the spine) of the shoulder blade. You can feel this muscle on both sides simply by shrugging your shoulders straight up and holding for a second. This muscle is an almost universal site of constriction and tension and can cause pain in the neck and shoulder, as well as irritate the "trigger points" in the other neck muscles, resulting in headaches.

Most shoulder pain is caused by tendinitis, tendinosis or bursitis, or by arthritis or direct injury. Symptoms include swelling in the shoulder area, pain during movement or after periods of inactivity, stiffness, or a feeling that the shoulder isn't "tracking" properly. Most shoulder pain results when muscles, tendons and/or ligaments in the shoulder area are injured or overused.

Tendinitis is an inflammation of the tendons and tissues surrounding the shoulder, usually caused by injury or overuse. Similarly, excessive or repetitive use of the shoulder can also lead to bursitis (see last section). When pain persists after inflammation has gone, it usually indicates the more common and somewhat more serious condition known as tendinosis.

A common reason for shoulder pain is degeneration or injury of the rotator cuff, a group of tendons that attach the upper arm bone with the shoulder blade and facilitate the raising and rotating of the arm.

General Injury to the Neck

Strain

Muscle strain, also known as a "pulled muscle," can be anything from a slightly overstretched muscle to something more severe like a torn muscle or tendon – therefore symptoms can vary from annoying to misery-making. Depending on severity, symptoms can include pain and tenderness that is worse with movement of the neck and/or shoulders, swelling, limited range of motion, burning and, when a tear is present, actual bulging at the site of the injury. When the injury is minor, the pain typically goes away after a few days, but as we know, ignoring even simple neck strain can turn it into an "onset event" that will create a cycle of recurring problems. More severe cases of neck strain absolutely demand adequate treatment, including gentle stretching, support-building exercises, massage and **TENS** treatment to loosen tightened muscles and increase circulation.

Sprain

A sprain is a stretch or tear in the ligaments that connect the bones to one another. They can range in severity from first to third degree, third degree being the most serious. The injury known as "whiplash" is one example of a sprain to the ligaments of the neck and upper back.

- **First-degree sprain:** *the ligaments stretch but don't tear. Symptoms may include moderate swelling, mild to moderate pain, some stiffness in the neck and upper back and headaches.*

- **Second-degree sprain:** *the ligaments experience a partial tear. Symptoms may include feeling or hearing a "pop" at the time of injury, moderate to severe pain – particularly in the posterior neck muscles, swelling or bruising, restricted movement of the neck, a feeling of heaviness of the head, muscle spasm in the shoulder and headaches.*

- **Third-degree sprain:** *the ligaments are torn completely. Pain can be moderate or quite severe, though it is interesting to note that the pain may be less in a complete tear than in a partial one. Symptoms also include tingling, numbness, a "grating" sound or feeling when the head is moved side to side, severe swelling and a visible bulge in the neck or upper back at the site of the tear and headaches.*

Most neck sprains usually occur from an event such as an accident or a fall. Even if your sprain seems minor, you should be examined by your doctor to eliminate or identify concurrent injury such as spinal fracture, disc injury or dislocation.

Recovery time can be affected by your age, overall health and the severity of the sprain. A severe sprain can take months to heal and, as with any injury to the neck, can create ongoing problems if not treated appropriately to facilitate circulation, regain full range of motion, halt swelling and eliminate the buildup of noxious chemicals that an injury will release in the affected local muscles.

Whiplash

The syndrome known as "whiplash" is a general injury to the ligaments and muscles that support the cervical spine due to a sudden, jolting extension of the neck. Most people associate the term with a car accident, which is perhaps its most common cause, though it can also be caused by a direct blow that pushes the head forward very suddenly, such as being forcefully struck to the back of the head.

Whiplash can be excruciatingly painful, though its symptoms often don't show up until within two or three days following the injury. Symptoms can include any or all of the following: mild to extreme limitation of movement of the head and neck, pain radiating into one or both shoulders, arms and/or hands, and pain or numbness through the upper back between the shoulder blades. It can also cause maladies associated with poor nerve conduction or blood circulation to the head, such as severe and/or chronic headaches, dizziness, ringing in the ears, blurred vision, difficulty concentrating or remembering, irritability, insomnia and fatigue.

The most common treatment for whiplash is to render the neck immobile, typically with a cervical collar, until symptoms improve, but this is a treatment that is often over-prescribed. In fact, unless there is inflammation or unbearable pain, a collar may exacerbate symptoms by disallowing normal range of motion to help the body's soft tissues and joints get the circulation and "washing" movement they need in order to heal. Once movement is possible without too much pain, control and strengthening exercises and regular massage stimulation with a **TENS** device will help to increase circulation, heal the injured tissues and prevent segmental facilitation and other common consequences of this type of trauma.

Sports Injuries

Training, practice and competition are demanding on an athlete's body and can often lead to injuries both minor and serious. Athletes are also prone to repeat injuries because they often don't give themselves sufficient time for full recovery. While *types* of injuries are sport-specific, there are common elements to areas that get injured that can teach us how to achieve maximum recovery in the shortest possible time. By understanding the basic anatomy involved in common sports injuries, recovery will be faster, more complete and achieved with the least amount of permanent damage.

Tissues Prone to Injury:

- **Muscles:** *Muscle strain is the most common type of sports injury. Straining, pulling or tearing of muscles will cause the muscles to contract and become "knotty." Repetitive straining will cause* *fibrous scar tissue to develop within the muscle fibres. Strained muscles that are not treated properly will become chronically inflamed, shortened, constricted, tender to touch, weak, inflexible and slow to respond. Tense muscles impede blood and nerve circulation, which increases pain and slows healing.*

- **Tendons:** *Tendons attach muscles to bones. When a tendon becomes inflamed by "excessive loading" (pulling on the tendon by strained muscles), the onset of tendinitis can occur. Overstretched tendons are vulnerable to tears within the tendon tissues or at the point of bone attachment. Rigid and inflexible muscles will make a tendon prone to tearing and repeat tearing.*

- **Ligaments:** *Ligaments attach one bone to another. Ligament-sprain injuries, which can be complete or partial tears, tend to occur when a joint is displaced beyond its normal function or alignment. Ligaments need sufficient blood circulation for fast healing, so it's important to relax the local muscles to promote blood flow, eliminate local inflammation and nourish damaged ligament tissue.*

- **Joints:** *A joint is formed by two bones that move against one another. The end of each bone involved in making a joint is lined with a smooth coat of cartilage, and the joint space between the bones contains synovial fluid to lubricate the cartilage when the joint is in motion. Some joints are more complicated: for example, the knee joint has two cartilage discs within the joint space to cushion impact and to allow a complex range of movement. Injured joints become inflamed and painful and, if the injury persists, secondary arthritis can occur. Joint injuries quite often occur along with muscle strains and ligament sprains. All injured tissues must be treated properly in order for the joint to get enough blood flow and movement for maximum recovery.*

While some serious sports injuries may require surgery, most respond quite well to treatments that relax the adjacent muscles and stimulate nerve and blood circulation to the affected area so that the injured tissues can repair themselves and leave minimal scar tissue behind. The RICE method (Rest, Ice, Compression, and Elevation) is quite effective when applied to swelling tissues immediately following an injury and is continued until swelling subsides. Then mobility exercises, stretching, massage and **TENS** therapy will aid circulation and help to restore movement.

Degeneration Disorders

Herniated Disc

Intervertebral discs are structures that are firmly locked between the thirty-three interlocking bones of the spine's vertebrae. The discs are made up of a tough outer casing (called the capsule) and filled with a thick fluid designed to absorb shock and keep the spine flexible. By as early as age twenty the discs begin to flatten, even with normal wear, and their "jelly filling" (called the nucleus) starts to dry up and become less shock-absorbing. Injury, overuse or repeated misuse can encourage the development of tiny tears in a disc's capsule and allow the fluid inside to break through, creating a herniated (also known as ruptured, slipped or protruded) disc. In spite of the commonly used term "slipped disc," there is really little room for spinal discs to slip or move. What actually happens is a disc's inner material is leaking through the rubbery outer membrane and placing pressure on the surrounding nerves.

When a disc in the neck herniates, it may bulge or leak enough fluid to cause enough pressure on the spinal cord or nerves to lead to weakness, numbness and pain in the head, arms and hands. Herniated discs are one of the prime causes of pinched nerves (see below). Although a jarring injury can damage a disc, most problems seem to be brought on by everyday activities – improper lifting, falling or making a sudden, uncontrolled movement. It has also been estimated that as many as 70 percent of cases are a result of poor posture placing constant pressure on the vertebrae, which then causes a herniation or leaves the discs vulnerable to outside injury.

You will probably find it interesting to learn that as we age and the inner material of our spinal discs hardens, we become less susceptible to disc herniation, since the inner fluid has a lesser likelihood of "oozing" outside its capsule. The greatest number of reports of the problem occur in men under fifty, possibly because they are young enough to attempt grandiose movements and just old enough that their discs don't appreciate the exertion.

One way to test the discs in your neck is to try this exercise: clench your hand into a fist as if you're about to knock on a door and pull your arm backward. If you can't do it without pain, it's possible that a disc in your neck is causing nerve pressure. The only way to know for sure, of course, is to have your doctor perform an examination and perhaps an imaging test such as an X-ray, CT scan or MRI.

Luckily, in most cases a herniated disc can be managed simply by allowing tears in the capsule to heal. In order to encourage healing, however, it is important to know the cause. If the problem appeared immediately after an injury then the cause is probably obvious. If it appeared "out of nowhere," then you must take an inventory of your history of injury: did you have a car accident or a fall?; did you suffer any blunt-force trauma to your head, neck or upper back?; did you attempt to catch a heavy falling object? If you can remember no such incident, even one from years ago, then you must consider your posture as a possible culprit, including the posture you take when you sit, stand, use the phone, sleep and do activities that require you to hold your arms in front of you (including cooking, typing and driving) or over your head (like painting or construction work) for extended periods. For more information on posture, see my brief discussion of the topic in the "Treatment and Prevention" chapter.

Standard medical treatment for a herniated disc is often surgery and, in my experience, surgery offers little long-term relief for most people. So how do you treat a herniated disc? In the vast majority of cases, a ruptured disc will heal itself with appropriate home treatment. As with many other spinal disorders, herniated discs involve tightly contracted muscles and scar tissue surrounding the affected area. This chronic muscle tension causes pressure on the degenerated disc and worsens the protrusion and pain. Chronic muscle tension will also restrict full joint movement and deprive the joint surface of the lubricating and nourishing synovial fluid it needs to stay healthy. By utilizing treatments that relax the muscles and relieve the pain, you can simultaneously remove pressure to the affected disc, which will often reduce the protrusion and pain and allow beneficial movement needed for the body to repair the damage.

Pinched Nerve

When a disc's inner "jelly" gets pushed through its tough outer casing, or when a piece of the capsule itself breaks off, it can "strangle" any of the nerves exiting the neck. The same effect can be caused by bone spurs, spinal stenosis and other disorders.

More commonly, however, pinched nerves are caused by pressure exerted on them by tense, inflamed muscles alongside or around them. When surrounding tissue presses against a nerve and interferes with its function, it can result in aches, pain, numbness or a weakening of the affected muscles. Many things can cause a pinched nerve – injury, repetitive movement, joint disease, poor posture, even pregnancy . . . Though pinching can happen to almost any major nerve in the body, among the most commonly affected are those extending through the shoulders down the arms to the hands.

Pain, numbness and/or weakness will often be felt not only where the nerve is pinched, but also in the destination point of the irritated nerve. A pinched C7 nerve can cause an arm and hand to ache or go numb. A compromised C6 nerve will cause the shoulder to ache or be "frozen" and difficult to lift. The key signs that you suffer from a pinched nerve are numbness and weakness, either residual or constant, whether or not they are accompanied by pain. Some patients report that they frequently wake up with one arm and/or hand numb (or as they usually put it, "asleep") suggesting that their sleeping posture or pillow is causing a cervical nerve to become pressed. The best way to relieve a pinched nerve is to remove the tension from the muscles that support it and increase circulation to the area. Once this is achieved, provided the nerve is not being pinched by a hard object such as a bone spur, the numbness and pain will disappear.

Osteoarthritis

The most common form of arthritis, osteoarthritis (also called *degenerative joint disease*) is associated with a breakdown of cartilage in the joints and commonly occurs in the cervical spine. OA is often split up into "common degenerative arthritis," the variety that evolves from the wear and tear of ageing and to which we become more susceptible as we grow older, and "secondary osteoarthritis," which can affect people of any age and arises from previous injuries. Any kind of injury to a joint – whiplash, a fall, an overexertion or overuse injury – can begin the process of secondary osteoarthritis. **OA** develops slowly and usually affects more than one joint at a time: the joints of the neck, fingers, wrists, shoulders, spine, hips, knees, ankles and toes are most prone to the condition, which causes the cartilage in a joint to stiffen and lose elasticity, making it more vulnerable to injury or damage. In some joints the cartilage may actually wear away over time, causing tendons and ligaments to stretch and become painful. If cartilage continues to erode, the affected bones may actually rub against each other. Symptoms of **OA** include:

- *Aches and pains in joints, especially during activity.*
- *Pain during or after overuse.*
- *Extreme stiffness and/or pain after long periods of inactivity, especially in the morning.*
- *Mild to moderate swelling of certain joints, especially of those in the fingers.*

In my experience, **NSAID**s provide only limited and temporary relief and are often overused by people suffering from **OA** pain. The best and most health-supporting treatments for pain include employing hot and/or cold compresses, gentle stretching, exercise and massage therapy (including **TENS** therapy) to the affected areas to provide relief, increase circulation and prevent further degeneration of the joint cartilage. Also important is implementing proper weight control, since **OA**'s symptoms seem to be worsened by excess body weight.

Rheumatoid Arthritis

Rheumatoid arthritis is a chronic inflammatory disease that mainly affects the synovial membranes of several or many joints in the body, usually in a "mirrored" fashion – meaning that inflammation usually strikes identical joints on both sides, such as both shoulders or both middle fingers. RA's symptoms include severe swelling, redness, pain and stiffness and can occur in any of the joints of the body, most frequently in the wrists, fingers, elbows, knees and ankles.

RA, which affects women three times more often than it does men, can begin at any time in one's life, from childhood to adulthood – in adults its onset is usually between the ages of forty and sixty years. RA is generally more serious the earlier it begins, because over time it can lead to joint malformation. It is considered an autoimmune disease, in which a person's own immune cells attack the joint tissue and genetic factors appear to play a role. The HLA-DR4 antibody, as well as antibodies to IgG, both considered to be rheumatoid factors, are present in roughly 70 percent of adult patients who have the disease, suggesting a genetic predisposition.

Most RA patients experience remissions and exacerbations of their symptoms, meaning that there are usually good days and bad. Sometimes a patient may have so many good days that they believe their RA has gone into full remission. Full remission does happen, but it is uncommon and therefore vitally important that anyone who has RA continues the treatment program established by his or her specialist; feeling "cured" means that your treatment is working and should be sustained. RA can be aggressive and will progress quickly if correct treatment is ignored or discontinued.

The causes of RA are widely and vigorously studied but, thus far, inconclusive.

As with OA, I find the greatest relief comes from gentle exercise, mild stretching routines such as yoga, massage and **TENS** therapy to increase range of motion and improve joint function.

Arthritis in the Hands

Many people get arthritis in the hands. Arthritis *can* be associated with ageing, but if you start getting hand arthritis that isn't related to either ageing or a form of systemic arthritis such as rheumatoid arthritis, then once again you'll probably be able to trace your ailment back to your neck. If the nerves there are not conducting properly, the body's daily repair process will be impaired and, over time, early joint degeneration can occur. It is quite common for this degeneration to spread downward, causing the previously described symptoms in the shoulders and elbows, and finally to affect changes in the fingers – making knuckles and finger joints start to look and feel enlarged. For many, osteoarthritis, the arthritis we typically link to the elderly, can be a result of poor neck function, which begins the process that eventually leads to an arthritic change in a distant joint such as a finger joint – it gets stiff, looks swollen, becomes enlarged and feels painful. And again, I'm not talking about people in their sixties and seventies; a lot of people I see with this condition are thirty to fifty years old – a range we don't normally associate with arthritis. For them and others with arthritis of the hands, massage and **TENS** treatment of the C7, C8 and T1 nerves will almost always provide the best and most dependable relief.

Spinal Stenosis

Spinal stenosis is arthritis of the spine. It can be considered a normal part of ageing, but in recent years the condition has become more common in younger people due to overuse injuries that act as onset events for arthritic change, or from simple disuse of the neck causing the ligaments around the cervical spine to become inelastic and thickened.

As the intervertebral discs lose their water content and begin to compress, bone spurs may appear and press on spinal nerves, causing pain, numbness and weakness that radiate into the upper extremities (as well as lower limbs if the arthritis extends into the thoracic and/or lumbar sections of the spine). Cervical stenosis can create pain that limits neck and head movement, and the subsequent inactivity worsens the degeneration and the symptoms associated with the disorder, including aching, tingling and burning, or reduced sensitivity in the neck, shoulders, arms, hands and fingers. Compression of the cervical nerves can also create headaches, dizziness and fatigue.

Increasing the conductivity of the cervical nerves is important in preventing further degeneration of ligaments and muscles in and around the neck. Promoting proper blood flow is vital in helping the body's tissues to heal their daily tears and fissures and prevent worsening of the arthritic condition. I have found that the best ways to maintain strength and motion are regular exercise, a gentle daily stretching routine, massage and TENS therapy.

Cervical Spondylitis

Cervical spondylitis is a mechanical disorder that most often occurs in people over fifty, in which chronically stiff neck muscles cause the cervical spine to crook forward. As with other modern-lifestyle, early-degeneration maladies, however, it is more frequently occurring in younger people, far sooner than it should. In most cases, **cs** is caused by poor posture and a lack of exercise taking their toll over time, bringing about spine malformation. Staying hunched over a computer, bending to perform a task such as assembly work, sleeping with your head propped too high or tilted to one side, or sitting for long periods with your head against a headrest - such as those on luxury office chairs and in your car - can force the cervical column into an unnatural forward position that bends the spine. This direct pressure on the bones and cervical discs can lead to damage such as curvature of the spine and bone spurs.

The most common symptoms of **cs** include neck pain that sometimes radiates down the arms to the hands, numbness in the fingers and headaches from neck-muscle tension. Typically sufferers report that the trapezius muscle at the back of the neck and upper back is tender and full of knots. This constant tension in the trapezius irritates the nerves of the cervical spine and can cause compression of the upper spinal cord, which may in turn cause serious symptoms including pain in the brachial plexus (felt around the collarbone and chest), the upper extremities and the shoulder blades. The pain can become so bad that it makes even simple movement agonizingly difficult.

The best treatment of cervical spondylitis is proper ergonomic support, including good posture that relieves pressure on the cervical spine, a pillow that supports proper spine alignment, regular exercise to keep the trapezius muscle strong and loose, and massage and **TENS** treatment to relieve tension, improve circulation and flush waste products from tight muscles.

Spasmodic Torticollis

Quite often babies arrive with their heads twisted to one side, a condition called *congenital torticollis* that, left untreated, can turn into an "onset event" that will leave the child vulnerable to neck dysfunction later in life. Massage and very gentle stretching can treat congenital torticollis and prevent any permanent damage it might cause to the child's range of motion.

Spasmodic torticollis is a less common, chronic condition that affects approximately three people out of every ten thousand. ST is a movement disorder caused by brain dysfunction, and it can cause intermittent or sustained neck muscle contraction that causes the patient's head to lean to one side or tilt forward or backward. It may cause the person's shoulders to sit unevenly and is quite often very painful, limiting a person's ability to function during the course of the spasm.

There is no standard treatment for ST, but people I've treated often respond well to a combination of physiotherapy and electrical muscle stimulation using a TENS device morning and night, a routine that can release the muscle spasm and allow the patient to regain control of his or neck function.

Notes:

Migraine and Tension Headaches

Headaches are something that practically every one of us has experienced at least once in our lives – most of the population will endure some grade of headache from once a week to once a month. In fact, it is estimated that headaches cause between 5 and 10 percent of young adults to miss at least part of one workday each month – an alarming statistic.

The causes of headache are many, from common and frequently overlooked sources like mild dehydration, to those less well-known, like food allergy. Headache pain is so prevalent that it is included in over fifty percent of the complaints that people take to their doctor's office. American Medical Association research suggests that 90 percent of headaches are classified as being caused by muscle tension, meaning that even though they are agonizing, they are not pathogenic or necessarily chronic. Only about 6 percent are migrainous in nature, with the remaining four percent falling into the mixed or rare categories. The pathogenic causes of headaches, such as cerebral aneurysms, tumours, strokes, TIA (transient ischemic attacks), meningitis or encephalitis are comparatively rare, but please note that anyone suffering from severe, unexplained or unremitting headaches, or a headache that is accompanied by other symptoms like blurred vision or vomiting, should see a doctor to rule out such possibilities.

This chapter will deal with the standard and less serious types of headache – tension, cervicogenic (relating to your neck) and migraine – and a couple of less common causes such as **TMJ** (temporal mandibular joint) disorder and sinus pressure caused by allergy or infection. Headaches can vary remarkably in severity, triggering factors, location, frequency and duration. The intensity of headaches can range from a dull pressure behind the eyes to a constant throbbing or stabbing pain behind one or both eyes, temples, or in different areas of the head such as the top, side(s) or brow bone. For most people, headaches typically have a gradual onset and last anywhere from a few hours to several days, and then gradually abate. Many people relate the onset of a headache with emotional stress, such as excessive worrying, anxiety or anger. Some people experience headaches only a few times in their lives; some endure them every day. One thing all headaches have in common is that they make you suffer: a mild headache can make simple tasks more difficult and limit concentration; while a severe one can force you straight to bed.

In my nineteen years of practice it has been my experience that almost all headaches, from mild to chronic, can be effectively managed and in many cases prevented from recurring through a combination treatment program of massage therapy, exercise, good posture practice and relaxation/breathing techniques. For example, let's look at the case of one of my patients:

Louise is a fifty-eight-year-old woman who suffered from migraine and tension headaches for over thirty-seven years. Her headaches were often so severe and disabling that she felt sick to her stomach and was unable to do anything but rest in a dark room. Any stress, noise or light tended to aggravate her agony. Her head pain is located at the left temple and frontal region of her head. She complained of pain in the left temple and frontal region of her head, and of severe pressure and a stinging sensation behind her left eye, both occurring two to three times per week in headaches that could last the full days. Her usual treatment included taking pain medications prescribed by her neurologist and family doctor. The medications would not alleviate the headaches completely but they did reduce the intensity of the pain. However, the medications caused her to feel drowsy and weak and gave her concern about the potential long-term side effects the medication might have on her health.

Electroencephalogram (EEG) and X-rays did not reveal pathology.

Upon physical examination of her neck, we took note of a tenderness at the rear upper area just below her hairline, but no other significant findings.

I recommended that she use Dr. Ho's Muscle Massage System on her upper neck for eight weeks. She treated her neck at least three times per day – when she first woke up in the morning, after dinner and again before bedtime. She also used the device on her upper neck when she felt a headache coming on. She reported having only one headache over the first week of treatment. The intensity was mild and she did not need medication. In fact, she immediately used the device on her upper neck and the headache ceased after fifteen minutes. By the third week she was free of headache pain and reported that she felt much more energetic and clear of mind. She continued with the daily treatments for the eight weeks as recommended, and after that only as needed when she felt a headache coming on. Louise tells me that she now enjoys life more because she no longer has to make plans around her disabling headaches. She feels secure that whenever a headache threatens, she has the tools and knowledge to manage it.

Classification Of Headaches

Generally, I put a low priority on trying to classify headaches other than as pathogenic or non-pathogenic. Naturally these are important distinctions because disorders that are pathogenic, or caused by disease, can be serious, even life-threatening. But as for the vast majority of headache causes, I prefer to look at the symptoms, and then use them to construct a list of the possible causes or aggravating factors. Classifying non-pathogenic headaches won't make them go away any faster, but for most sufferers, curiosity about what is causing their pain invites a certain amount of classification, which I will address here.

Pathogenic Headaches

Pathogenic headaches are usually easy to identify because they're so uncommon. The most serious causes are tumours, cysts, aneurysms (balloonings or leakages of a blood vessel in the head), subarachnoid hemorrhages (bleeding caused by direct injury, infection or vascular malformation) and intracranial swelling caused by diseases such as meningitis. A less serious cause can also be glaucoma. Headaches associated with the serious causes can include other distressing symptoms including dizziness, extreme sensitivity to light and/or noise, nausea, vomiting, fainting, loss of vision and others. Pathogenic headaches can strike a person who never gets headaches without warning or reason – no triggers and no aggravating factors. Pathogenic headaches often very closely mimic migraine headaches in both severity and symptoms, so anyone who has a "first time migraine" should see his or her doctor immediately for a diagnosis.

Doctors usually refer patients showing symptoms of pathogenic headache directly to a neurologist for a CAT (computerized axial tomography) scan, an EEG and/or MRI for a better look at the problem. I've done this for a few patients in the past as a precaution, but none of them tested positive for a tumour or any other life-threatening disorder – as stated before, such events, thankfully, are uncommon, but never to be ignored.

Non-Pathogenic Headaches

Non-pathogenic headaches include tension headaches, cervicogenic headaches, migraine headaches, TMJ-disorder-related headaches, sinus headaches, menstrual headaches, headaches caused by dehydration, by medication, or by food allergies, and "combination" headaches. Let's start with the most common:

Tension Headaches

Tension headache is a rather vague title for a very common problem. Since 90 percent of headaches are diagnosed as tension headaches, you'd think the medical community would have a complete and solid understanding of what the term means. But the term *tension headache* actually meets with a lot of resistance among healthcare practitioners. The Ethic Committee of the National Institutes of Health opposes the term in favour of the phrase *muscle contraction headache*, because the committee believes that the word "tension" implies a possible emotional cause. They believe that *muscle contraction headache* is more medically accurate because it specifically suggests tension of the pericranial muscles, which are those that cover the skull.

Frankly, I find the debate to be rather fruitless. The medical community often tries tirelessly to divorce the physical and the emotional pillars of health, which I see as impossible. Anyone who has ever been in agony will tell you that pain can bring out negative emotions. Any depressed or angry person can tell you that negative emotions are often accompanied by physical reactions. Tension creates tension: a bad day can cause your muscles, including those covering your skull, to tighten and, left untreated, to stay contracted. Pain creates its own physical tension - press a sore spot and your first reaction is to flinch, which is nothing more than an immediate contraction. Whether your body is "flinching" because it is retreating from physical or emotional discomfort (or both) isn't the real issue as far as your body is concerned. It is merely utilizing its rather crude alarm system to signal that something is amiss.

Everyone reacts to stress differently, and different muscles can tense in response to it. Some people get tense in the abdomen, some people get tense in the lower back and others carry a lot of facial tension. When muscles in the head, such as the *temporalis* (temple) and the *frontalis* (forehead) tighten, they can cause the discomfort that constitutes the classic medical definition of a tension headache. Another type of tension headache, however, is caused by tension of the neck muscles. It is called the *cervicogenic headache*.

Cervicogenic Headaches

Because the neck is already one of the tensest areas in the body, many people react to stress by creating muscle tension there. Once the muscles become contracted, they can irritate the upper cervical nerves, C1 and C2, which send pain signals to the nerves in the head, and *voila*, a headache is born.

How do these nerves get irritated? Unfortunately, it's quite easy.

Let's once again take a quick look at the cervical spine. The head sits atop the first vertebra, called the *atlas* after the Greek god who balanced the world on his shoulders. The atlas looks sort of like a small plate and acts as a platform on top of the pivoting second vertebra, the *axis*. Directly alongside these vertebrae, all the way down the back of the neck and into the upper back, is the trapezius muscle. As the occipital nerves that exit the atlas and the axis enter the trapezius, they become instantly vulnerable to any pressure or spasm that this large muscle endures. Muscle tension, or any other restriction of free movement of the joints, discs or ligaments anywhere along the path of the trapezius, can lead to nerve irritation. This irritation can in turn cause reflex muscle spasm and produce continuous tension in the neck muscles (segmental facilitation). Tension headaches, whether initiated by physical tension caused by, say, poor posture, or emotional tension such as holding in your anger at your boss, are the result of sustained neck muscle contraction that producing nerve irritation and direct pain from *ischemia* – restricted circulation and subsequent lack of oxygen – within the muscle tissue itself.

Irritation of the C1 and C2 nerve roots (which are often accompanied by irritated C3 and C4 nerves) on their paths from the spinal cord to the occipital muscles at the base of the skull can result in pain to the head. In my experience the C1, or suboccipital nerve, is the most common culprit. When this nerve gets irritated, it can cause anything from a mild pain to recurrent migraine-like symptoms: pressure behind the eyes and in the sinus cavity, throbbing at the temples at one or both sides, or sharp pain that people sometimes describe as feeling like being stabbed with a hot poker. And for some, these symptoms occur on a regular basis – weekly or even daily.

Severe headaches can cause sufferers to feel tired all day long, from the moment they awake to the time they go back to bed. Often people report having a tight band-like pressure across the forehead and behind the eyes, sometimes accompanied by dizziness and/or insomnia. I spend much of my practice dealing with the C1 nerve when it has been irritated by tight muscles to create these disturbing symptoms.

For some people a cervicogenic headache is triggered by a little extra stress at work or at home. Or, it can happen every weekend, during changes in the weather, before or during menstrual periods or when people eat something that doesn't agree with them – a cervicogenic headache is easy to trigger. And the symptoms are often connected to migraines or other forms of headaches, the origins are almost always traced to the most common reason for headaches – nerve irritation in the neck.

Migraine Headaches

Migraine is an episodic disorder that can be so serious that it interferes with one's quality of life. If your doctor has diagnosed you as having a migraine headache, you've probably exhibited some common signs and symptoms: severe stabbing or throbbing pain over the temple area – typically on one side, pressure behind the eyes, sensitivity to light and/or noise and oftentimes nausea and vomiting. And sometimes there are pre-headache signs, such as seeing black dots or spots of light, what we call *scotoma*, or feeling a cold sensation, that tend to occur just before major head pain comes on. People displaying these medical-textbook symptoms of migraine headache will almost always be diagnosed as having a migraine even when they don't. Truthfully, many people can have these symptoms with a tension or a cervicogenic headache. And often the migraine diagnosis invites the headaches to repeat themselves because of the stress and expectation of misery that has been mistakenly placed on the sufferer, who now believe him/herself to be a *migraineur*.

Migraines are a vexing problem for the medical community, because they're not well understood and often expensive to treat. It is reported that more women suffer from migraines than men, but the data is inconclusive because it may be that women are simply more willing to seek treatment for recurrent headaches. It is true, however, that hormonal fluctuations such as those associated with menstruation can bring about a migrainous episode, which may make women more regularly prone than men.

Migraine headaches can be triggered by a lot of things, such as weather changes, the menstrual cycle or the intake of certain foods, but most of the time they seem to come for no reason at all.

Traditional treatment almost always involves prescription medication to help prevent the onset of a migraine attack and, that failing, something to help relieve the agony once it arrives. Some people find that certain medications do help prevent the frequency of their attacks, but often these work for a limited time before losing their efficacy. Few people in my experience get substantial relief from medication designed to treat the symptoms once they arrive. In fact, many people unknowingly suffer from headaches brought about by overuse of pain medication. It is important to note that as many as 86 percent of migraine patients *overuse* medication, so a substantial number of headaches may be a consequence of simple overdosing. Also notable is that caffeine, which most migraineurs believe helps relieve their suffering, is a frequent contributing factor of headache pain.

I've found that many migraines begin in the same source spot at tension and cervicogenic headaches - the C1 (and sometimes C2) nerve(s) in the upper neck - and can be prevented by treating those areas directly. For many of my patients, daily **TENS** therapy reduces the frequency of attacks and in some has managed to all but eliminate them. In almost all cases, the need for medication is drastically reduced, diminishing not only the adverse impact that such medications have on the body's internal organs, but also the headaches that these medications frequently produce.

TMJ (Temporal Mandibular Joint) Headaches

TMJ is a disorder of the temporal mandibular joint. You can locate the temporal mandibular joint simply by placing your finger just in front of your ear and opening and closing your mouth - you'll feel the joint create a small cavity as your jaw opens. Some people suffer **TMJ** disorder because their upper and lower jawbones are misaligned or because one the two is over- or undersized. However, some **TMJ** sufferers are simply people whose posture, misuse of the jaw and/or emotional stress affects their jaw mechanics.

If you think back to the last time you were truly angry but couldn't express it (the most common version I hear regarding this kind of repression is toward one's boss, for obvious reasons), you may remember clenching your teeth. If you try it right now, you'll feel the muscle at your jaw line bow out – this muscle attaches to the temporal mandibular joint and supports its movement. You can also stress this area by eating hard food that is too large for your mouth (this is where the candy "jawbreaker" gets its name), or having something that alters your bite – such as braces, dentures or dental implants. Even something as simple as keeping your mouth open wide for a prolonged time, such as during dental work, can create serious tension in the jaw muscle. This tension, whatever its source, is another common cause of head pain and headaches. If you have any pain radiating from that area upward, you can be fairly sure that you have a **TMJ**-related headache. This category can also be mistaken for a migraine due to its trait of producing severe pain near the temple at one side of the head.

Sinus Headaches

As many as thirty-five million people in America alone suffer from sinusitis, a general term referring to any kind of inflammation or irritation of the sinuses. Inflamed sinuses don't drain properly, causing pressure within the sinus cavities that can create headaches. Interestingly, the forward cavity in your head known as the *nasal cavity,* which connects directly to the nose, is not part of the sinus even though sinus pressure is often felt there. The sinuses, which are divided into left and right halves, include the *frontal sinus,* which sits above your eyes just behind the forehead; the *maxillary sinus* located on either side of the nose just below the eye and above the upper teeth and extends to the back of your throat; the *ethmoid sinus,* which sits between your eyes; and the *sphenoid sinus,* which resides far back in the head behind the eyes and the nasal cavity. This sinus is just in front of the brain, making any complications here serious, but luckily these are rare.

The sinuses work to keep the body free from germs and other alien matter by fighting them off at the first point of entry past the nose. Germs that these cavities fail to conquer can enter the body and create disease and infection. Hence, the main source of sinus infection is stuffiness or drainage in the collection area of bacteria and viruses itself: the nose. The sinuses are irritated by any excessive foreign matter they encounter – even harmless elements like pollens, grasses and other airborne substances, making them inflamed and creating pressure that can be felt around the nose, eyes, head and brow bone.

However, many people who have pain in the sinus region don't necessarily have sinusitis. I've found that if the C1 nerve is irritated, a cervicogenic headache can present itself in the sinus area through the nerve connections between the upper cervical nerves and nerve endings embedded in the sinus cavities. As a result, many patients are prescribed antibiotics unnecessarily for sinus headaches because the cause is presumed to be sinus infection, when in fact they have undiagnosed neck problems. True sinus infection produces not only facial pressure and pain, but also other symptoms such as congestion, discoloured nasal discharge or nasal obstruction, and occasionally fever.

Providing you don't have any of these other symptoms along with your headache, it's unlikely that you have a sinus infection and likely that treatment of the C1 nerve will alleviate the pain.

Menstrual Headaches

Many women report getting severe headaches during or just before their menstrual cycle begins. Menstrual headaches are usually cervicogenic or migrainous in nature and can occur two to three days before or up to five days after the onset of menstruation. The rapid hormonal fluctuation can cause bodily and emotional stress that the body instinctually reacts to with muscle contraction. The upper neck muscles are already tight, so when the body undergoes premenstrual or menstrual stress, these muscles actually contract even more – enough to irritate the C1 nerve and trigger a headache.

In my practice, I've been able to confirm that irritation of C1 is the cause of most menstrual headaches, because once we treat the problem by relaxing the neck and upper shoulder muscles, and by loosening up the exit joint and getting the nerves properly circulating, most patients no longer get headaches associated with their menstrual cycles. However, true migraine headaches can also be brought on by menstrual periods that somehow interfere with the autonomic nervous system (the body's "automatic" or "self-controlling" nervous system), which directs blood flow to the head area. This condition is considered a true migraine headache because the menstrual period is related to neurohormonal changes that affect the blood circulation in the head. Even in cases of true migraine, however, treatments designed to increase circulation to the head, such as massage and TENS treatments, can often help prevent headaches and reduce the pain and duration of one that has already arrived.

Headaches Caused by Allergy, Dehydration and Medication

The food allergy headache is typically a migraine or cervicogenic headache. Certain foods, such as wheat, nuts, chocolate, artificial sweeteners, ingredients in red wine and in cheese, and MSG (monosodium glutamate) in Chinese food and in products like Accent, are among many known to cause blood vessels to contract or dilate. They can all trigger migraine-like headaches in some patients because contraction of blood vessels in the head often causes pain – this process is a true food-induced headache. Sometimes, though, a food allergy is another source of stress on the body that causes the neck to tighten up more than usual and prompts a cervicogenic headache. If you keep a diary of your headache episodes, you may notice that you react to certain foods to which you may have an allergy. If you notice that you get headaches within the minutes or hours after ingesting, say corn, you may have an allergy to it. The best thing to do is cut out each possible allergen one at a time and stay off it for two weeks. Then try reintroducing the possible culprit back into your diet. If your headache recurs, you should avoid that food entirely.

Another very common cause of headache (in fact, one of the most common) is simple dehydration. You get busy and forget to drink enough water, or you drink too much caffeine or alcohol or eat too little food – all causes of dehydration – and you can quickly get a headache. As often as a drug like Aspirin "cures" a headache, the mere act of ingesting water to wash it down can be what helps to alleviate the pounding in one's head. A hangover is nothing more than a more pronounced version of the dehydration headache, and anyone who has ever had one knows how horrible they can be. But many people suffer from a less pronounced form of dehydration every day – they simply don't drink the 64 oz. of water that the body requires to flush its toxins effectively. Yes, you should drink a minimum of eight 8-oz glasses of water per day, which may seem like a lot, but it is actually a normal amount for the average body. A good rule of thumb is to take note of the colour of your urine: if you notice that it is distinctly yellow or golden, then you're dehydrated. By drinking enough to ensure that the urine you expel is clear, you can prevent dehydration headaches altogether.

And, as mentioned before, over-medication can easily cause headaches. Any of the NSAIDs such as Aspirin, ibuprofen (Advil), naproxen sodium (Aleve) and others we use to relieve headaches can cause what are known as rebound headaches, the body's response to overexposure to the medication. Overuse of even Tylenol can cause a headache response, not to mention the myriad of other herbal, over-the-counter and prescription medications that we take for *other things* that can inspire a headache to erupt.

Combination Headaches

Oftentimes the actual causes of a headache are not simply one thing, but a combination. As many as 64 percent of people with migraines, for example, are thought to suffer headaches that are a combination of migraine, tension and medication overuse. Or, a headache can easily be brought on by a combination of hormonal fluctuation and dehydration, or by neck muscle tension from driving in heavy traffic compounded by the emotional stress of arguing with your spouse. In order to achieve the most complete recovery from a headache, it's important to examine and identify all the possible aggravating factors and eliminate them wherever possible. Certainly eliminating traffic or your moody teenager is not an option. But recognizing the stressors in your life, both physical and emotional, and limiting them or removing them is the key to preventing headaches. Also important, no matter what type of headache plagues you, is to loosen up the muscles in your neck and get the nerves to your head flowing properly. It seems that no matter what type of headache people endure, loosening the neck muscles through gentle exercise and massage can offer at least some relief. And for people with muscle tension and cervicogenic headaches (which is most of us), it can offer great relief.

CHAPTER FIVE

Fibromyalgia and How to Treat It

Fibromyalgia is such a perplexing and life-altering disorder that it and its treatment rightly deserve a full chapter. If you or someone you know suffers from this disease, I hope you'll take the time to read this section to better your understanding of the syndrome and the suffering it can cause. I have treated many patients with FM and I can tell you that you're not alone.

What is Fibromyalgia?

Fibromyalgia (FM) is a chronic condition associated with widespread pain in the body's soft tissues (muscles, tendons and/or ligaments), fatigue and other symptoms. Its name identifies it directly: "fibro" meaning fibrous tissues, "my" meaning muscles and "algia" meaning pain.

A common complaint of patients with fibromyalgia is that they ache all over, as though their muscles are strained or as if they have the flu. The disorder can cause patients to sleep poorly, be stiff upon waking and feel tired all day. Some patients also experience other unpleasant symptoms such as frequent headaches, muscle spasm, dizziness, numbness, tingling, abdominal cramping, even problems with memory and concentration.

FM's side effects can vary in severity from day to day and migrate from one muscle location to another, often focusing on areas used most often such as the neck, shoulders and feet. In some people, the pain can be so intense that it interferes with even the simplest movements, while in others it may cause only slight discomfort. The associated fatigue of FM also varies widely among patients, ranging from a general feeling of tiredness to utter exhaustion.

Certain factors, such as changes in the weather or relative humidity, cold or drafty environments, hormonal changes, stress, depression, anxiety and fatigue can all contribute to symptom flare-ups, though often they occur for no identifiable reason.

What Causes Fibromyalgia?

Fibromyalgia is a diagnosis that can feel like a prison sentence. No one truly understands the cause of the disorder and the theories that the medical community has offered to explain it don't include enough evidence to be considered definitive proof, so FM remains a mystery. Some possibilities include the following:

1. **Increased sensitivity of nerve cells.** *It is one theory that FM sufferers have an advanced sensitivity of the central nervous system, which is composed of the spinal cord and the brain. Because the central nervous system extends to the peripheral nervous system (the nerves that branch out to the rest of the body), widespread muscle pain is FM's primary symptom. This increased sensitivity may cause a hyperactive brain/body response to basically normal stimuli (allodynia) or a magnified response to real pain stimuli (hyperalgesia). In either case, the*

pain restricts movement and the suppressed movement creates stiffness.

2. **An imbalance of brain chemicals.** *Some people may inherit an anomaly in the way their brains regulate and produce certain neurotransmitters, including substance P, which notifies the body of pain experiences and is found in abnormally high levels in FM patients. Perhaps compounding the problem, the neurotransmitter serotonin, which modifies the intensity of pain signals entering the brain, appears to be deficient in sufferers of fibromyalgia. Because serotonin is regulated during sleep, however, it is difficult to say whether it is deficient due to lack of sleep or if sleep deprivation causes it to become deficient. Over time the sleep deprivation creates widespread pain in the muscles and soft tissues, making movement difficult. In support of this theory, similar symptoms, such as muscle pain and tender points can be produced in people who do not have FM simply by depriving them of deep sleep for a few days.*

3. **An imbalance of hormones.** *During sleep, the pituitary gland releases a specific cocktail of hormones responsible for maintaining good muscle and soft tissue health. When they get out of balance it can cause decreased energy, pain in the muscles and joints, water retention, irritability and insomnia.*

4. **Deficient growth hormone.** *A reduced level of growth hormone has been associated with fatigue, muscle weakness, increased sensitivity to cold and a reduction of memory, among other problems.*

5. **A traumatic triggering event.** *FM may have triggering events that lead to its onset, such as a serious viral or bacterial infection,*

an auto accident or the development of another disorder such as rheumatoid arthritis. These triggering events probably don't cause FM, but rather, they may awaken a hidden genetic predisposition.

6. **Decreased oxygen.** *Another possible cause supported by clinical studies is poor muscle oxygenation, meaning some muscles are not getting enough oxygen. This simple lack of oxygenation is considered by many experts to be the reason the soft tissues become so contracted and racked with pain. Contracted muscles not only cause the brain to release chemicals that can heighten pain, they're too tight to allow in enough oxygen, creating decreased fluid levels in soft tissues, a limited ability to repair injuries and a cycle of misery.*

Any (or none) of these theories may pinpoint the cause of FM. Because the syndrome mimics other soft tissue disorders, patients who have symptoms but show no laboratory abnormality are often concluded to have fibromyalgia, since FM causes pain but not swelling, heat or redness. It also produces no traits visible in X-ray or blood tests.

Truthfully, the medical community is utterly confounded by fibromyalgia, and this confusion often leads to incorrect diagnosis, either missing FM as the reason for pain or concluding that someone with a different illness has FM. It also leads some MDS to suggest that FM is a psychosomatic disorder: that is, one that the patient creates out of mental conflict or stress. If you have read my section on Tension Myositis Syndrome (TMS), you know that emotional conflicts can and do create very real physical suffering and damage, and deserve an equal amount of respect in their treatment. But in my experience, patients with FM are not people whose emotions create their painful condition. Certainly emotions created by having the disease can worsen one's symptoms and should be addressed, but the fallback of "blaming the patient" for his or her malady is one I find inappropriate in this case, even insulting. If you or someone you know has FM, it's important to understand that it is a disorder with *physical* origins, but whose symptoms carry over into the emotional realm, as is true of any ongoing physical problem. Who among us is at our most pleasant and productive when we're in pain? The pain is usually the strongest focus of the brain, and life's small problems and victories quickly take a back seat.

Regardless of its cause, fibromyalgia perpetuates a vicious cycle of *increased* sensitivity to pain and *decreased* physical activity. One symptom worsens the other until both become unbearable, leading to chronic fatigue, poor sleep, sore muscles and a decreased ability to repair muscle damage.

In spite of both the medical community's and the general public's lack of knowledge about FM, it is actually fairly common. It is estimated that roughly ten million Americans and Canadians (about 2 to 4 percent) suffer from fibromyalgia syndrome. Most are women between the ages of twenty-nine and fifty years old, but it can happen in either gender and to people of any age and race. It can occur after a serious illness, trauma or injury or begin gradually over time with no known incident. FM often runs in families (similar to chronic fatigue syndrome and migraine headache), suggesting it may be an inherited trait.

Believe it or not, there is some good news about fibromyalgia. In spite of its being a very unpleasant condition that produces painful side effects, it is not a degenerative or deforming disorder and does not interfere with a person's lifespan or overall health. In fact, with proper treatment and a dedication to a healthy lifestyle, many of FM's symptoms can be reduced dramatically and allow you to live life to its happiest and fullest.

The Symptoms of FM

This list of major symptoms of FM is for your reference – it is not intended to diagnose fibromyalgia, which should be left to a doctor familiar with the disorder. If your regular doctor, or even a specialist you may be have been referred to, seems inadequately versed in diagnosing and treating FM, investigate doctors in your area until you find one who knows the disease forward and backward. If you need help locating one, try contacting a local FM support group and ask for recommendations. You'll not only get a personal recommendation from someone who has a first-hand understanding of your issues, you'll also meet others who share your concerns. Support groups can be a great way to help deal with the stress of both FM as well as all the mishaps life deals us – an important component of treatment.

Testing to determine if you have FM requires a very specific series of steps and will probably take an hour or longer – it's not a disorder your doctor can identify just by hearing your symptoms. An FM specialist will first ask if your pain has been present for at least three months and if it is widespread across your body (in all four body quadrants: upper and lower, left and right). He or she will then perform an examination called the "Tender Point" test in which approximately four kilograms (about nine pounds) of pressure are applied to specific points within the following areas:

1. *Neck area (below the hair line).*
2. *Sides of neck.*
3. *Upper shoulders.*
4. *Shoulder (rotator cuff).*
5. *Front of the chest.*
6. *Outer elbow.*
7. *Upper third of the buttock.*
8. *Posterior hip joint.*

9. *Inside of the knee joint.*

The American College of Rheumatology guidelines suggest that a true case of fibromyalgia will produce at least eleven "tender points" out of a possible eighteen on the sites listed above (nine on each side of the body). The reason FM may not be diagnosed with fewer painful sites is that its symptoms so closely mimic other illnesses or injuries that occur commonly across the population. For this reason, it is important that you seek an informed professional before jumping to conclusions.

If you suspect you may have FM but haven't yet been diagnosed (or don't have faith in a diagnosis you've been given), I recommend keeping a health diary and noting any of the following (or other) symptoms you may be experiencing, including their frequency and time(s) of day that they occur, so you can aid your healthcare provider in correctly determining your condition and its treatment:

1. **Pain:** *The pain of fibromyalgia can be wide and varying. One patient may experience a deep muscular aching or burning, while another may complain of throbbing, shooting or stabbing pain, either mild and intermittent or deep and constant. Quite often the pain and stiffness are at their worst in the morning and in the muscles used most commonly, like the neck and shoulders. Unlike the pain commonly associated with arthritis, FM's pain can move from one body part to another, affecting the back one day or hour and the feet the next. It is important to note that in order to be considered pain associated with FM, it must occur both above and below the waist, on both sides of the body, cause tenderness in key areas (see the list), and it must be present three months or longer.*

2. **Fatigue:** *Again, this symptom varies widely from patient to patient. Some experience mild fatigue (often associated simply with the poor sleep that accompanies FM) and others are so exhausted they have trouble getting through the day, as if they have the flu. The fatigue of FM is sometimes called "brain fatigue," leaving its sufferers drained both mentally and physically. This exhaustion may make some people feel lethargic and as if their limbs are too heavy to move. Similarly, they may have trouble concentrating as if they are sleep-deprived — even if they have had plenty of sleep.*

3. **Sleep disorders:** *Research suggests that fibromyalgia sufferers usually have an accompanying sleep disorder called the alpha-EEG anomaly (the same anomaly associated with chronic fatigue syndrome). The research found that FM patients typically fell asleep without much trouble, but their deep sleep was regularly interrupted by atypical rapid brain activity. Patients appeared to spend much of the night in "half sleep," as if they were somehow fully asleep and yet wide-awake at the same time. This causes FM patients to wake up unrefreshed in spite of having slept the whole night through. FM patients may also have other sleep disorders, such as teeth grinding (bruxism), sudden nighttime jerking of the arms and legs (myoclonus), periodic leg movement (PLMS) and restless leg syndrome (RLS), which is characterized by a "creepy crawly" sensation in the legs and an irresistible urge to move them when at rest or when lying down. Needless to say, any of these can be very disruptive to the patient as well as to his or her sleeping partner and can contribute to feelings of exhaustion.*

4. **Gastrointestinal Problems:** *Irritable bowel syndrome, nausea, abdominal pain, cramping, bloating, constipation and/or diarrhea*

are common complaints associated with FM.

5. **Chronic headaches:** *Roughly half of FM patients also report migraine or tension headaches. While the association is not clearly understood, it definitely adds to the suffering of the patient.*

6. **Temporomandibular Joint Dysfunction Syndrome (TMJ):** *TMJ produces mild to severe face and head pain in one quarter of FM patients — in most FM patients, however, the discomfort is thought to be related to the muscles and ligaments surrounding the joint and not necessarily the joint itself, as with true TMJ.*

7. **Increased Headaches, Facial and Shoulder Pain:** *Roughly half of FM patients also experience head, facial and/or shoulder pain (myofascial pain syndrome or MPS), often as a result of very stiff or sore neck and/or shoulder muscles. MPS produces "trigger points" in the neck, shoulders and jaw that can be very painful and can radiate pain to related areas of the body.*

8. **Chemical Sensitivity:** *About half of FM patients report increased sensitivity to chemicals including fragrances and cosmetics as well as household cleaners and other products. They may also have reactions that mimic allergies, like itching, rash, nasal congestion, runny nose or sinus pain (but do not produce the measurable immune responses that allergies do) to a variety of substances that don't bother most people.*

9. **Sensory Sensitivity:** *Some patients report being abnormally sensitive to light, sound, touch and odours, which some medical professionals attribute to hyperactivity of the nervous system. Some people with FM say they feel chilled or hot when others*

around them are comfortable.

10. **Dysmenorrhea:** *Many women suffering from FM complain of painful periods, including menstrual cramps and abdominal pain, diarrhea and/or constipation.*

11. **Cognitive Disorders:** *FM patients may experience feeling "spacey" or as if they are "in a fog." They often report having problems remembering simple nouns or people's names and may feel overwhelmed when engaging in more than one task at the same time.*

12. **Genitourinary Problems:** *FM patients may experience an increased need to urinate, or a false sense of urgency – a symptom that mimics that of a bladder infection. Some women with FM may also suffer from conditions such as vulvar vestibulitis or vulvodynia, characterized by a painful vulvar region and/or pain during sexual intercourse.*

13. **Paresthesia:** *This term refers to the numbness, tingling, prickly feeling or burning that occurs in some FM patients.*

14. **Chest Pain:** *Individuals with FM who engage in certain activities like typing, sitting at a desk or doing anything that requires long stretches of forward body posture often have complaints about chest and upper body (thoracic) pain, shallow breathing and/or posture problems. They may also develop a condition known as costochondralgia (also known as costochondritis), referring to pain where the ribs and the chest bone meet. Costochondralgia is often mistaken for heart disease because of the location of the pain. However, if you are an FM patient and you have chest pain, please never presume it is the FM causing it – contact your*

physician immediately to rule out more serious causes.

15. **Problems with Equilibrium:** *Because fibromyalgia may affect the tracking muscles of the eyes, you may experience blurred vision, dizziness and nausea whenever you are visually tracking anything, as with driving a car, reading or watching a ball game. In addition, trigger points in the head or neck may cause dizziness or loss of equilibrium. Research conducted at Johns Hopkins Medical Center also suggests that some FM patients may have "neurally mediated hypotension" which causes a drop in blood pressure and heart rate when they stand up – resulting in light-headedness, nausea and difficulty thinking.*

16. **Skin Complaints:** *Some FM patients experience itchy, dry or blotchy skin. Others may experience the sensation of swollen limbs, fingers or toes, even though swelling itself is not a symptom of FM. These strange feelings may also be attributed to the theory that FM involves a hyperactive nervous system, but for now the distinct cause is unknown.*

17. **Depression and Anxiety:** *Because FM can be difficult to recognize and diagnose (it produces no "evidence" that will show up in an X-ray or blood test), many FM patients are told that their symptoms are caused by depression or anxiety disorders or even hypochondria. While it is true that stress can exacerbate symptoms of FM, there is no evidence to suggest that it is its cause. It is important to note that FM's symptoms may by their nature produce feelings of depression or anxiety, as is true with any health concern. It is vitally important for people suffering from FM to monitor and treat these conditions, as they can interfere with successful symptom management.*

As if the list provided in this book isn't enough, there are still other symptoms of FM I haven't touched upon. Fibromyalgia's symptoms are vast and varying (and many are common symptoms caused by other things). Yours may not have been addressed, so make sure to keep detailed notes of any symptom that might relate to your condition and provide them to your doctor.

Treatment of FM

Some of the treatments for FM, such as relieving pain in specific areas of the neck, shoulder and upper back – which account for nearly half the tender points in FM patients – you will find in the general "Treatment and Prevention" chapter. But since FM produces so many pain sites, to keep things easy and to expand to other sites of pain beyond the neck area, I have included a special section here just for those who must deal with FM's particular problems.

Treatment of Specific Tender Spots

The following list describes common tender or painful regions associated with FM and how they cause some of the symptoms experienced by patients. Understanding the cause and relationship of different symptoms is important in determining the type of care that will offer optimal relief.

1. **Suboccipital region.** *This is the area at the back and upper part of the neck, just below the hairline and about one inch from the midline on both sides. The tender point is in the depressed region where the suboccipital muscles are, specifically where the*

suboccipital (C1) nerve exits between the bottom of the skull and the first vertebrae of the neck. Unknown to most patients with FM, irritation of this nerve can cause headaches, migraines, fatigue, insomnia, dizziness, the inability to concentrate and feelings of pressure and stabbing pain behind the eyes and temple region. Upper neck muscle tension, tenderness and associated symptoms will typically worsen just before or during menstruation, during sleep and with emotional or postural stress.

Relief: *Try to avoid activities that strain the neck muscles. Proper integrated massage and specialized daily neck exercises in the morning and just before bedtime are necessary to relieve the suboccipital muscle tension and to restore the circulation of the C1 nerve. Regular neck massage or use of a TENS device such as Dr. Ho's Muscle Therapy System along with exercise can re-educate these neck muscles to stay relaxed and pain-free.*

2. **C5, C7 transverse process area.** *This area can be felt about 1.5 inches from the midline at the sides and lower back of the neck. When tensed and chronically contracted, these muscles cause neck pain and restriction of movement that is worst in the morning and after prolonged sitting. They can enter into spasm, causing more acute neck pain, in response to emotional stress, poor posture and during sleep. Unknown to most patients with FM, tight muscles in the sides and lower back of the neck will cause irritation (***thoracic outlet syndrome***) of the brachial plexus nerves that exit the side of the neck and travel down the shoulder, through the elbow and wrist into the hand. Many patients with FM also suffer from unresolved elbow pain (***epicondylitis***,* **tennis** *or* **golfer's elbow***), or a recurrent*

*numbness and indescribable tingling feeling (**paresthsia**) deep in the arm and hand (if left untreated, the hand can lose strength and coordination over time).*

Relief: *Massage or apply a TENS device such as Dr. Ho's Muscle Massage System on the lower neck, upper back, forearm and wrist area on a daily basis to relax the tensed muscles and to stimulate the nerve circulation from neck to hand. Specific exercises should be performed three to six times per day in order to restore neck and upper shoulder movement.*

3. **Trapezius muscles.** *These tender spots are located on both sides at the midpoint of the crest of the upper shoulder muscles. Most FM patients will have several tender spots or zones of tenderness on each side. Chronic tightness of the trapezius muscles will cause the muscle fibres to harden and noxious chemicals to be released. Combined with poor circulation, the tightness will also cause a burning sensation that is both physically and emotionally distressing. Chronic FM patients are often highly emotionally sensitive due to chronic fatigue and constant pain from their muscle tension, pain and stiffness.*

Relief: *A combination of massage or use of a TENS device such as Dr. Ho's Muscle Massage System, muscle strengthening, and deep breathing relaxation exercise will help to keep tense muscles relaxed and pain-free..*

4. **Supraspinatus and rhomboid muscles.** *Often described by FM patients as an achy spot just beside the shoulder blade, in most cases this ache emanates from the upper back area between the shoulder blade and the spine – either on one side or both sides. Aside from being much deeper than the other*

tender spots, this pain often sharply radiates up to the head and neck area. It can be related to the **rhomboid muscle**, *which connects the scapula (shoulder blade) to the spine, or the* **supraspinatus muscle** *that connects the scapula to the humerus (arm) bone. This local tenderness and sharp pain may also be associated with the* **costovertebral joint**, *which is the connecting point between the rib and the spine, and may explain why some FM patients have corresponding chest pain at the* **costochondral junction** *on the side of the sternum (breast plate).*

Relief: *Massage or apply a TENS device such as Dr. Ho's Muscle Massage System on the rhomboid muscles, the supraspinatus muscles and the neck muscles daily. Specific exercises should be done daily to ensure good upper body posture and proper movement of the rib cage.*

Pain Relief Exercises:

For supraspinatus muscle pain, try the windmill motion exercise for the shoulder. Hold one arm straight up in the air. Clench your hand gently into a fist. Swing your arm down forcefully enough that it will move all the way around in a large circle back into the starting position. While the arm is going back up, let it go completely loose for the momentum to carry it back up. Repeat ten times and then go the opposite (backward) direction ten times. Three key things to remember with this exercise are:

- *Always start with the fist pointing straight up*
- *Swing downward as hard and as fast as you can*
- *Let your arm go completely loose and use the momentum, not your muscles to swing your arm back up.*

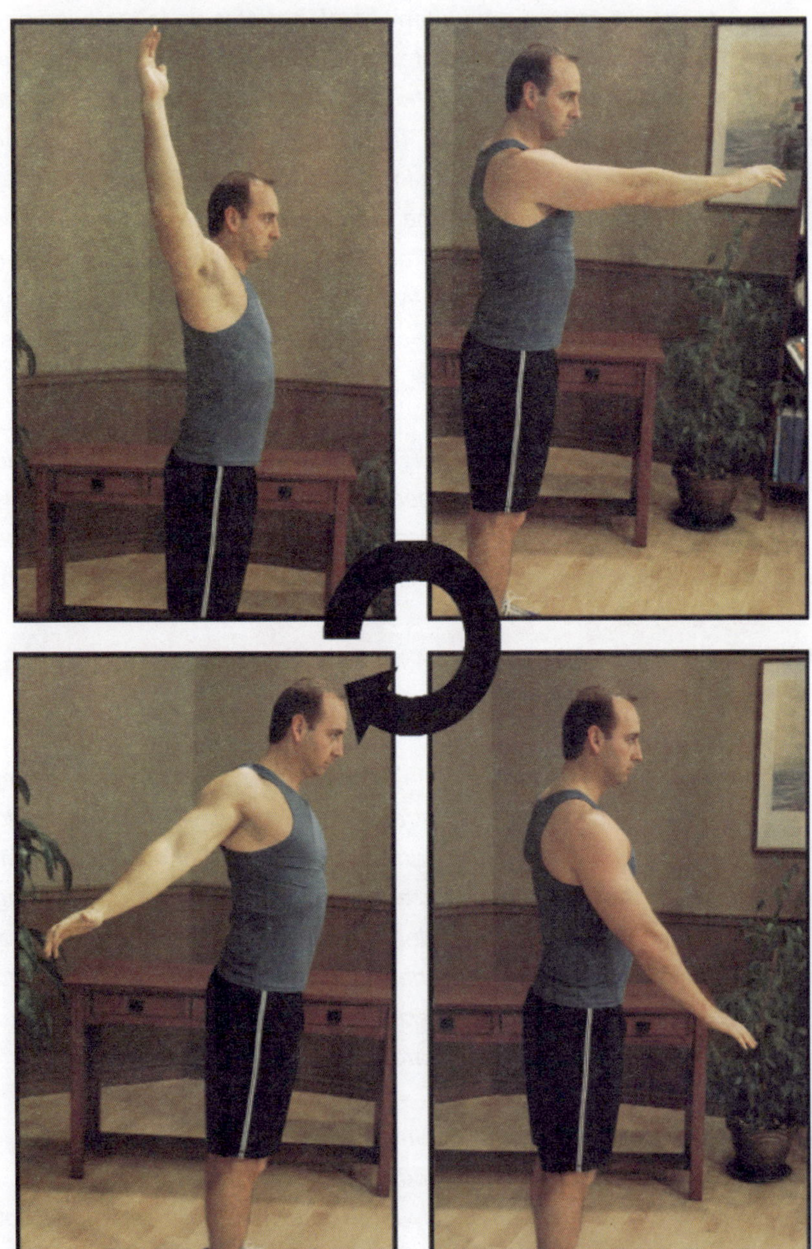

For pain in the rhomboid muscles and supraspinatus muscles, the best exercise to relax and add strength is push-ups. For most of you who have not done push-ups since grade school, start by doing standing bench push-ups.

Standing bench push-ups: Stand with evenly placed feet about three feet away from a solid counter. Place your hands about shoulder-width apart on the counter. Start doing ten push-ups two to three times per day. When you can do thirty standing bench push-ups without too much effort, progress to knee push-ups.

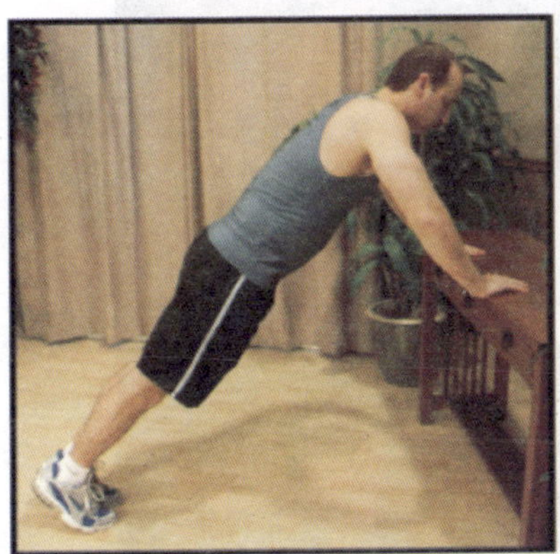

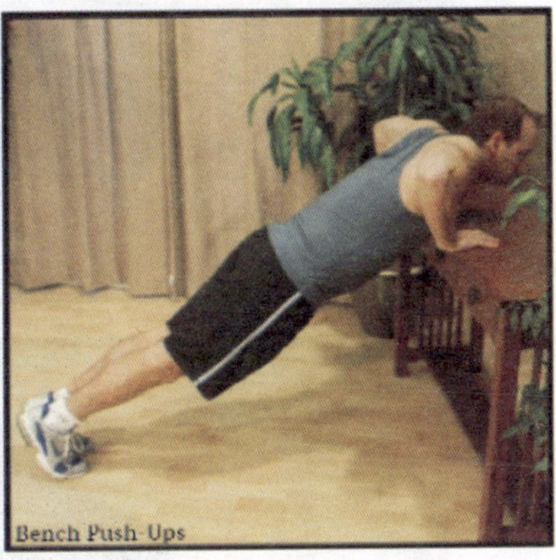

Bench Push-Ups

Knee push-ups. Begin with your knees and hands on the floor. Keeping your back straight throughout, start by doing ten push-ups two to three times per day. When you can do thirty without straining yourself, do regular push-ups with your legs fully extended, balanced on your toes.

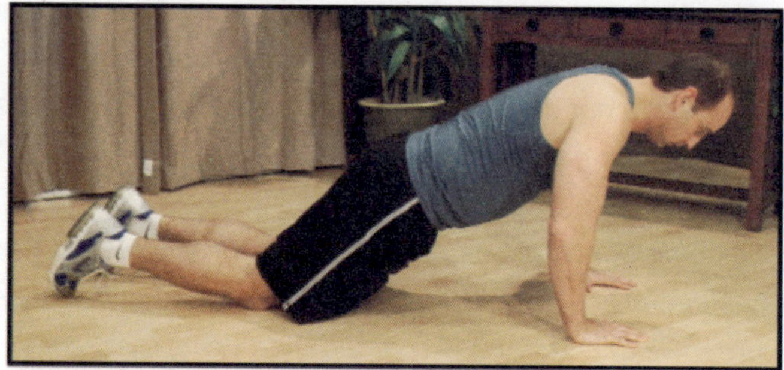

Knee Push-ups

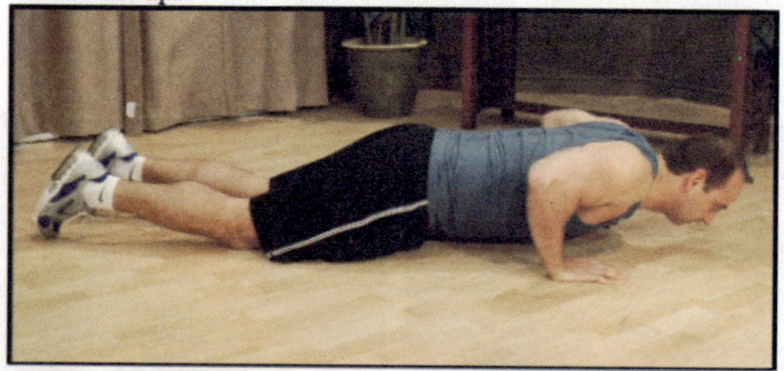

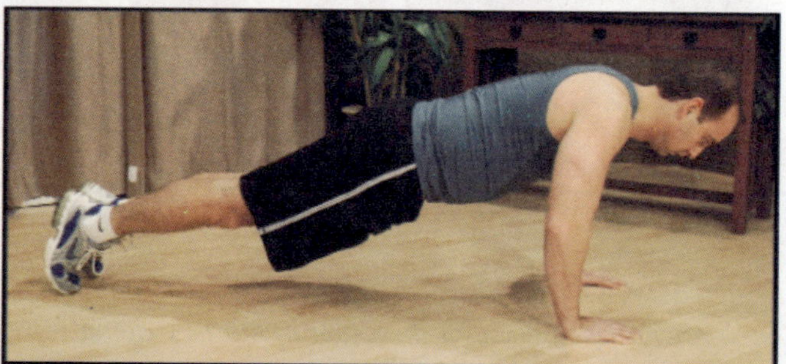

Toe Push-ups

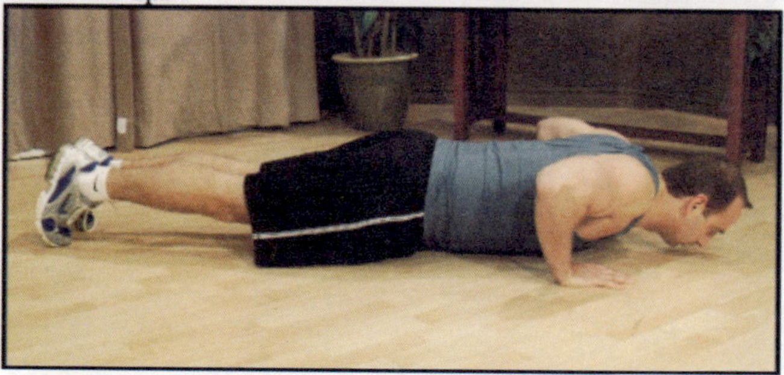

5. **Costochondral junction.** *This tender spot will situate itself at the front of the chest, over the joint connecting the rib to the sternum. It is common for the tenderness to be centered specifically at the level of the second or third rib. Many FM patients make the incorrect assumption that this sensation is due to an anxiety attack or a heart attack (though if you suffer this pain for the first time, see your doctor immediately to rule out other causes).*

   Relief: *Massage or apply a TENS device such as Dr. Ho's Muscle Massage System at the tender spots on the chest and the back of the shoulder blade area will often relieve the chest pain. Regular exercise to ensure good posture and a mobile rib cage will also help to keep the pain away.*

Pain Relief Exercises:

To treat pain in the costosternal and costovertebral joint, you will need to restore the motion of your rib cage by doing air push-ups. Standing air push-ups: Stand tall and point your fingers toward each other. Extend your arms in front of your chest as if you are doing a push-up against the air. Exhale fully as you push out. Now bring your elbows back and squeeze your shoulder blades together. Inhale deeply to expand your rib cage. Do ten repetitions. Repeat this exercise every hour throughout the day.

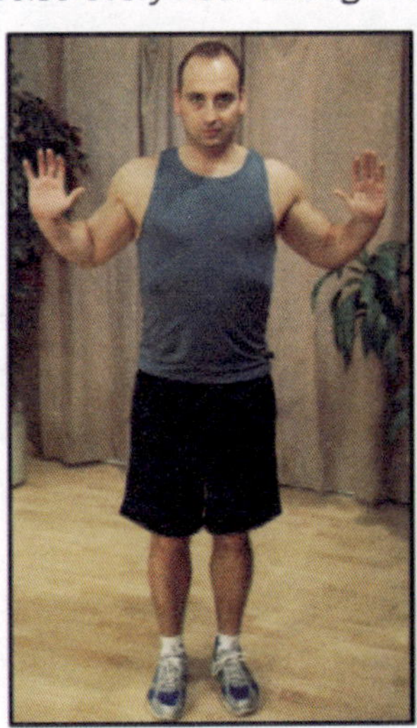
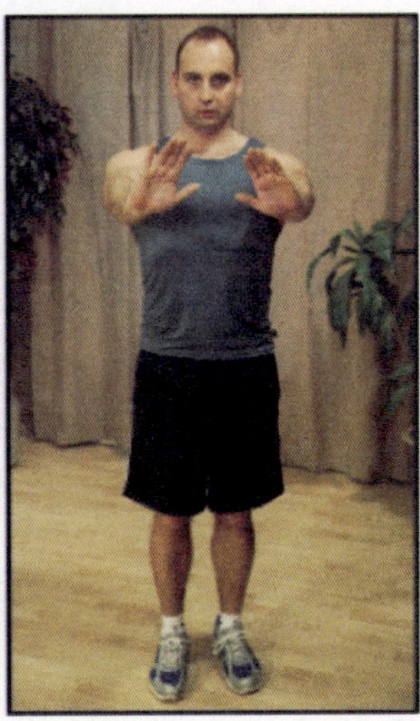

6. **Lateral epicondyle.** *This pain and tenderness, afflicting the side of the elbow, is often referred to as "***tennis elbow***". The pain is exacerbated with any forceful gripping or twisting hand motions. You may or may not have a history of elbow-overuse, as it is often related to poorly circulating brachial nerves that run from the neck to the elbow and hand.*

Relief: *It is very important to treat the neck as well as the elbow. Massage or use a TENS device such as Dr. Ho's Muscle Massage System on the forearm and neck muscles every day to teach them to relax again and to promote nerve and blood circulation to the elbow. Avoid any heavy work involving strong gripping of the hand or twisting of the wrist.*

7. **Greater trochanteric prominence and lower back.** *This feeling of sensitivity troubles the lower part of the back at the level of the sacroiliac joint (where the pelvic bone joins the sacrum tail bone) and the side of the hip. The cause is extreme tightness in the muscles at the lower back and at the* **piriformis muscle** *deep-seated in the hip. This can also irritate the sciatic nerve to send radiating pain down to the hip, knee and toes.*

Relief: *Be sure to treat the lower back and hip muscles. Massage or use a TENS device such as Dr. Ho's Muscle Massage System on the lower back muscles, the piriformis muscle in the buttock area and the side of the hip. Be sure to massage these muscles in the morning, before bedtime and during periods of prolonged sitting or standing. Performing a lower back and hip muscle stretch exercise on a daily basis will also help to keep muscle tension and pain away.*

Hip and Lower Back Stretches: To relieve hip and lower back pain, lie on your back and then pull one knee up toward the opposite shoulder, hold for ten seconds and then do the same on the other side. Perform the knee-to-opposite-shoulder stretch each morning and before going to bed. Repeat ten times on each side.

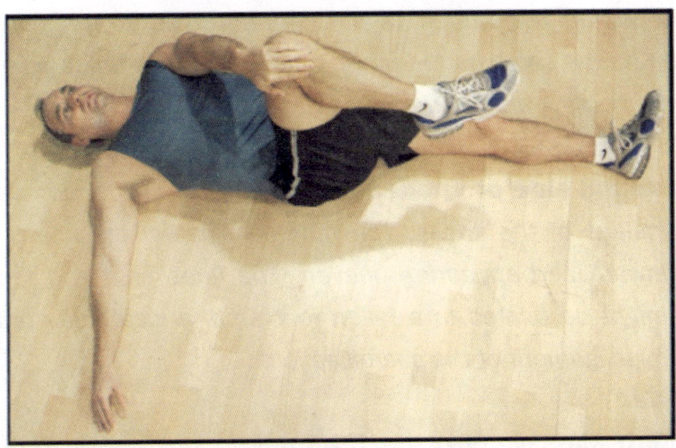

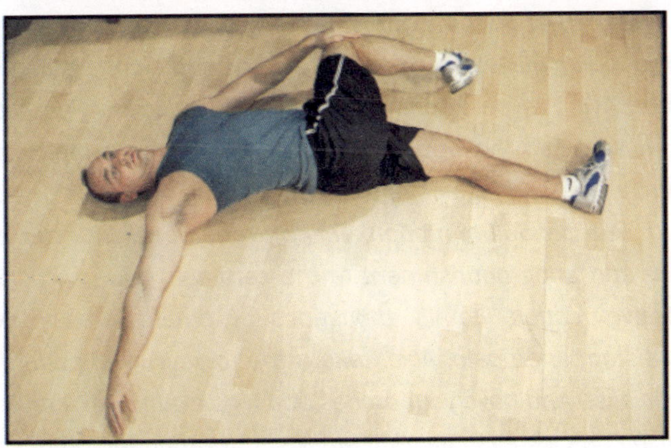

To stretch the hip, try the following: Lie on your back with your knees bent so that both feet are flat on the floor. Cross your right ankle over your bent left knee. Now lace your fingers behind your left thigh near your knee and gently pull your knee toward your chest. You will feel the stretch in your right hip. Hold for ten seconds and then do the same on the other side. Repeat ten times on each side each morning and before going to bed.

8. **Medial side of knee.** *Some patients report tenderness at the insides of the knees. You may also detect the knees pointing inward and appearing uneven. The knee pain and tenderness might be related to a fallen foot arch, a local knee problem or misalignment of the sacroiliac joint.*

Relief: *Massage or use a TENS device such as Dr. Ho's Muscle Massage System on both sides of your knee daily to relax the surrounding muscles and promote nerve and blood circulation to the area. Avoid hyperextending (locking) the knee. Passive motion exercises can be very beneficial: one I recommend is to sit comfortably in a high chair and gently swing your lower leg back and forth in a pendulum motion. This movement will lubricate the knee joint and bring nourishment to the cartilage. You can perform this passive motion literally thousands of times a day if you have persistent knee pain. Also, take a trip to your local pedorthist (foot specialist) and have your arches and legs examined. A fallen arch or having one leg even incrementally shorter than the other can cause pain in the knee(s), lower back, shoulders and neck. The right pedorthist can fit you with custom insoles to help correct the problem and take the strain off your joints.*

FM — The Body-Mind Connection

For maximum benefit, it is important for anyone who has been diagnosed with FM to take a whole body/mind approach to the treatment of its symptoms. Emotional stress may not cause FM, but it can contribute to its side effects and will certainly prohibit the success of any treatment. Poor physical health will obviously exacerbate the problems associated with the syndrome, so it is important for patients to do everything they can to relax their tight muscles, reduce emotional stress, establish and maintain regular soft tissue movement, and make every effort to establish good sleeping habits.

Let's go over a list of things to do to feel better now and during your whole life. You may be relieved to discover that most, if not all, of these recommendations could apply to anyone, for they are common-sense solutions and preventive measures for symptoms of illness, stress and injury:

- **Exercise:** *Regular daily exercise is key in regulating the growth hormone that maintains good muscle and soft tissue health and in assisting deep sleep. Since one of the major complaints of sufferers of FM is exhaustion, exercise is vital in helping to induce deep sleep and to limit restlessness. Many FM patients resist exercise and as a result carry excess weight, which can make symptoms worse. It's important to know that studies of FM patients show that any type of exercise is beneficial, from simple walking to gentle resistance training with elastic bands (such as Pilates equipment). Make it a priority and it will become easier over time and will reduce pain and insomnia.*

- **Be Aware of Your Limitations:** *Overdoing exercise or even laborious daily tasks will actually make your muscles contract — the opposite of what you want to accomplish — so start slowly.*

Your exercise should be vigorous enough to accelerate your heart rate, heat up your muscles and increase your oxygen intake and it must be sustained long enough to be beneficial. Your ultimate goal should be thirty minutes of aerobic exercise (or more if you feel up to it) every single day. Yes, daily, because exercise above anything else will help you to sleep, which is paramount to alleviating the symptoms of FM. Patients should stick to low- or no-impact aerobics such as brisk walking, bicycling (or stationery biking), swimming, or using a treadmill, stair climber or elliptical walking machine — any of which are available at most gyms. Strength training with elastic bands such as Pilates equipment has also proven helpful to FM patients.

- **Setting Goals:** *Reaching your fitness goal will take as long as your body and common sense allow. For some this regimen will begin with a walk around the block — listen to your body and don't push it beyond its limits. You should first consult with your doctor before embarking on your new fitness plan and even have him/her help you put one together that fits how you live.*

- **Stretching:** *Stretching exercises are very helpful in decreasing muscle stiffness and pain. When fibromyalgia patients have been immobile for long periods, for example upon waking or after sitting at a desk all day, their muscles tend to get stiff and painful. Stretching exercises and heat can be particularly helpful in alleviating these symptoms. There are videotapes available specifically designed to help FM patients do stretches correctly, to maximum benefit. Check your local bookseller or look online.*

- **Make Sleep a Priority:** *This is perhaps the most important component of treating your FM. It is important to try to maintain a regular sleep schedule, going to bed and waking at the same* *times. This schedule will help assist you in falling and staying asleep and feeling rested in the morning. If you have a partner who snores or a dog that barks or children who make noise early in the morning before you've had a chance to get a full night's sleep (and remember that a full night's sleep varies from person to person, from six to twelve hours a night), measures should be taken to make your sleep environment as peaceful and quiet as possible. Try to adjust the temperature of your sleeping environment so that you don't wake up stiff from being too cold or groggy from sleeping in an overheated room.*

- **Avoid Stress:** *"How can I avoid stress?" you may ask. What this involves is making yourself a priority when the need arises. Don't hang around people or in situations that make you feel bad, avoid situations that you find make you uncomfortable, don't take on more than you can handle. And if you find yourself experiencing stress (as we all do sometimes), take extra care to talk about it to someone you trust, go for a long walk, take a hot bath, exercise — whatever helps you to lessen the tension.*

- **Medication Where Indicated by Your Doctor:** *Your doctor may prescribe medication to improve deep sleep or to regulate the levels of hormones or neurotransmitters in your body. It is important to talk to him/her about your treatment and to seek a second opinion if your doctor seems to disregard your symptoms. Medication alone will probably not be enough to successfully treat FM, so it is important that you utilize it only as part of an overall healthy lifestyle commitment.*

- **Muscle stimulation:** *Specific electrical stimulation, or electrotherapy, of nerves and muscles can be effective in relieving muscle tension and pain. A specially designed device, called a TENS* *unit, stimulates the treated muscles to contract and relax with each electrical wave and feels relaxing, like a deep but gentle massage. Electrotherapy can help promote nerve conduction and blood circulation, relieving symptoms and greatly assisting the body's ability to heal. Proper devices feel good to use and do not create pain.*

What kinds of medications are used to treat FM?

A number of medications are used to treat fibromyalgia and depend primarily on the symptoms you display and your body's reactions. You and your doctor should work in tandem to decide which, if any, will best be used to treat your symptoms. Some include:

- *Desyrel (trazodone), an antidepressant.*
- *Flexeril (cyclobenzaprine hydrochloride), a muscle relaxant.*
- *Benadryl (diphenhydramine), a treatment for allergic symptoms.*
- *Xanax (alprazolam), an anti-anxiety drug.*
- *Soma (carisoprodol), a muscle relaxant.*
- *Elavil (amitriptyline), a sleep medication.*
- *Ambien (zolpidem tartrate), a sleep aid that can be used for a short term.*

Any of these medications can be used to induce sleep but they can cause unwanted side effects in some people, so it is important to share your concerns or reactions with your doctor before and during treatment. Your doctor will likely start you off at a low dose and gradually increase it until you're able to sleep through the night without daytime grogginess. It may be necessary to try out several medications or combinations before the right one is discovered. After two to four weeks of treatment most patients find that the treatment's side effects have lessened or disappeared and their fibromyalgia symptoms are starting to improve.

Other **FM** symptoms are sometimes treated by the following drugs:

- *Klonopin (clonazepam) and Mirapex (pramipexole), to treat restless leg syndrome (RLS).*
- *Neurontin (gabapentin) for nerve pain.*
- *Zanaflex (tizanidine hydrochloride) for muscle spasm.*
- *Prozac (fluoxetine), Paxil (paroxetine) and Zoloft (sertraline), to regulate serotonin levels, which has shown in some to alleviate pain.*

A new type of prescription drug known as a **COX II** inhibitor has also recently received **FDA** approval and been released on the market under the brand names Celebrex and Vioxx. Unlike other **NSAID** medicines, preliminary tests suggest that they carry a lower risk of gastrointestinal side effects. However, in spite of the misleading ads you might see on television and in print advertising, **COX II** inhibitor drugs are typically not indicated in the treatment of many people because they may increase the risk of heart attack, even in people under age sixty. Ask your doctor for complete details before using **COX II** inhibitors or any prescription medication.

Drug Interaction and FM

Some **FM** specialists suggest that it is important to avoid alcohol, narcotic sleep aids and those of the benzodiazepine group other than alprazolam (Xanax), since they may help you to fall asleep but will interfere with deep sleep, worsening your symptoms. Ibuprofen (Advil) does offer some people relief from pain, but it may cause sleep disturbances in some, so be mindful of your reactions to it. Ibuprofen can also cause gastrointestinal bleeding and ulcers, so it should be used in moderation. Acetaminophen (Tylenol) and the prescription medication Ultram (tramadol) have the least effect on sleep, but some may not find Tylenol offers enough relief from muscle pain. Ultram seems quite effective but can cause allergic reactions in some people, sometimes quite serious ones, so it is important to discuss its use with your doctor.

Herbal Remedies

Some patients report that they find herbal remedies helpful, even preferable over prescribed medications. As with any medicine, however, even herbal medicines should be investigated with the same caution and care you would use with any drug. Even herbal concoctions can have powerful interactions with certain medications, so discuss their use with your doctor.

Foods and FM

There has always been some controversy about whether or not diet has an affect on FM and its symptoms. But recent dietary research suggests that many FM sufferers are affected by diet, particularly by certain foods and additives.

Understanding which foods are the most health-supporting and therefore beneficial in dealing with FM's symptoms is fairly easy. It's the same sort of diet that doctors, dietitians and other health professionals have been advocating to the general population for years: unprocessed whole grain foods, fresh fruits and vegetables, and, if you eat animal products, small servings of lean, all-natural poultry and fresh fish. For example, it is a good dietary habit to eat at least two large servings of green leafy vegetables daily to ensure adequate fibre, vitamins, minerals and antioxidants for health. Some people naturally adhere to such a diet and for them keeping faithful to it is easy. For most, however, it is a real challenge.

When you're in pain and your options for enjoyment of life feel limited, food is an immediate source of predictable, easy and relatively inexpensive pleasure. A bag of Oreos, for example, costs only a few dollars and its rewards are instant: your taste buds thrill to the flavour and texture, your brain may react to the chocolate by releasing certain chemicals that make you feel elated for a few moments, and your belly feels nice and full afterward because of the high fat content. However, once the thrill is over (and it will be as soon as you take your last bite), you're left with the long-term woes of having eaten those cookies: the high calorie content will be difficult to burn off and your motivation to exercise will be low because your blood sugar soared and then crashed, leaving you feeling more tired that you did before. Even as you're tired, the caffeine in the chocolate will interfere with your night's sleep, compounding the insomnia that most FM patients endure; your arteries will have absorbed another incremental amount of sludge that over time can lead to many serious health problems; the high fat and sugar content as well as the "natural flavourings" (MSG) in the cookies will aggravate your symptoms and make your pain worse, not only today but tomorrow as well. And frequently such binges make people feel guilty and full of regret. So in eating those cookies you've sacrificed many aspects of your health and feelings of well-being just for a few moments of enjoyment. Unless it's a special occasion like your birthday, it will seldom be worth it.

Another important dietary element in preventing and lessening muscle pain – that will be easier for some than avoiding sugary snacks – is to drink at least 64 oz of fresh water every day (eight 8 oz glasses). Keeping hydrated helps to lessen muscle contraction by flushing noxious chemicals from the soft tissues, and keeps the organs free of the buildup of waste products, which can leave you feeling weak and under the weather. FM patients should consume the last of their water allotment about two hours before bedtime to avoid being awakened in the night by a full bladder.

Many patients report that certain foods, such as fatty, fried or sugary types, seem to invite or worsen fibromyalgia's symptoms. The reasons why are simple. Fatty foods actually temporarily "thicken" your blood, slowing the delivery of oxygen to your head and muscles. Less oxygen to your brain makes you feel tired, lethargic, even irritable; just as important, less oxygen to your muscles can make them ache, so the body pain that FM patients already endure becomes worse. Fried foods are very high in fat – the vast majority of the time in difficult-to-digest saturated fat, further adding to your symptoms. And sugary foods create massive swings in your blood sugar, which will rob you of the energy you need to keep moving to lessen your symptoms of pain, stiffness and insomnia.

Other people react to foods specific to their bodies, whether due to allergy or difficulty in digestion. Nuts, for example, may bother some and not others. If you suspect that some foods trigger your symptoms, try avoiding them and see if it helps. If you have trouble pinpointing which foods make you feel bad, begin keeping a diary of what you eat and how you feel in the hours following a meal or snack and eliminate those that may contribute to your discomfort.

For every FM patient, however, there are foods and additives that should be universally avoided:

- **Alcohol** – *alcohol spikes blood sugar levels, decreases energy and the desire to exercise and can exacerbate pain symptoms. And, in spite of the fact that it can make you sleepy, alcohol actually prevents deep sleep and will leave you feeling tired and* *dehydrated in the morning.*

- **Caffeine** – *even a small amount consumed in the morning can cause sleep disturbance. Be aware that many sodas and even some herbal teas contain caffeine, so it is a good idea to read the labels. If it doesn't boast that it is caffeine free, it is probably a good idea to assume that it isn't and avoid it.*

- **MSG** – *monosodium glutamate, which goes by a variety of names intended to disguise its use – including "natural flavouring," hydrolyzed vegetable protein and yeast extract – is in almost all processed foods. When MSG is broken down by the body, it can cause excited reactions in the spinal cord that can increase your sensitivity to pain.*

- **Aspartame** – *most recognized by its brand name NutraSweet, Aspartame is an artificial sweetener commonly found in sodas, candies, gum and other sugar-free or low-calorie processed foods. Studies suggest that FM patients often react to Aspartame with the same hypersensitivity to pain that is associated with MSG.*

- **Preservatives and Additives** – *highly processed foods (which include almost every convenience food in the market, from frozen food to boxed dinners to canned goods) contain preservatives and/or additives that can aggravate FM's symptoms, not to mention have an adverse impact on your health. Instead, eat whole, natural foods that have to be prepared at home. They'll be higher in flavour and fibre, lower in sodium and sugar, cheaper, and will provide you with greater energy and better health.*

- **Fried or Fatty Foods** – *these include obvious like fried chicken and Twinkies, but also the not-so-obvious like pork, hamburger and almost all dressings and sauces.*

- **Foods High in Sugar** – *sugar is hidden in many foods one probably wouldn't think of – including everything from salad dressing to french fries – so don't be fooled by processed foods that taste salty or tangy. Again, avoid processed foods and those high in concentrated sugars, including sugar, honey, molasses, fruit juices, cocktails, jellies, jams and ready-made sauces like spaghetti sauce.*

You may find yourself saying, "But Dr. Ho, you're asking me to give up all the foods that I love!" It may help you to know that I would give this advice to anyone I met in my office, whether they had FM or not. Good health is dependent to a large degree on eating well and exercising. You'll note that I never once said that you should go on a "diet" – diets typically lower people's blood sugar and make them feel weak, irritable and increase their pain symptoms. What I suggest is a complete eating overhaul. You'll not only feel better and have more energy, but those of you who may wish to drop some weight will find that it happens naturally – without hunger or complicated calorie-counting – and that you'll have a much easier time exercising and sleeping.

Doubtful? Try just two weeks of eating only whole, natural foods that you get from the health food store or the health food section of your local market. Eat lots of green, leafy vegetables, delicious peppers and other veggies that you enjoy, eat plenty of fresh tomatoes and grapes and other fruit favourites, and eat the whole grains that you prefer, providing you have no allergies. If you don't have reduced symptoms and feel better, you can always go back to your old ways. But my bet is you'll be surprised by how much better you feel – and look – after only two weeks. And if you stick to it for the long-term, your health and well-being will just keep getting better.

Alternative Therapies

As with all factors related to health, some things work marvellously for some and less so for others. What follows is a list of treatments and rehabilitation methods that have been helpful to some FM patients. You should pick and choose those you think might be helpful and discard those that do not prove to be effective for you.

- **TENS Therapy:** *TENS, which stands for Transcutaneous Electrical Nerve Stimulation, is a therapy in which electrical pulses stimulate muscle tissue, increasing blood and nerve circulation to treated areas. The stimulation allows the muscles to contract and then to expand, which helps to dispose of stored noxious pain chemicals, get blood to injured tissues and facilitate the relaxation of tense muscles. Many patients report that they experience pain and tension relief after their very first ten-to-twenty minute treatment. My study of TENS treatment led me to develop a device that offers more power, control and variety of stimulation than others on the market: Dr. Ho's Muscle Massage System.*

- **Massage:** *Most people respond positively to a relaxing massage. Massage can reduce stress, loosen tight muscles and increase circulation. If you are getting a massage for the first time or from a new practitioner, you should inform them of your fibromyalgia and work with them to find a pressure that will be relaxing and not so heavy that it causes you to tense up. Many therapists also provide heat and cold therapies to stimulate blood flow and ease tired muscles. If you find professional massage to be helpful but too expensive to utilize regularly, please see the massage section, which gives tips on how to teach yourself and those close to you* *how to provide relief at home.*

- **Chiropractic:** *Your chiropractor may be able to help loosen tight muscles and facilitate greater movement. Many people report that chiropractic methods offer them immediate and ongoing pain relief and greater flexibility. But it is important to use the same care in selecting a chiropractor that you would in choosing your regular MD; don't assume all chiropractic doctors are equally qualified to treat pain conditions. It is always best to get a recommendation from your MD or from someone you trust.*

- **Heat Therapy:** *Simple as it is, heat is a great way to relax aching or stiff muscles. Unlike arthritis, which involves inflammation and can be aggravated by heat, FM pain often responds very well to it. A hot shower or bath, sitting in a hot tub or spa, or applying a heating pad to sore muscles can provide immediate drug-free relief. Some people also report getting relief from "heat-producing" sports ointments like BENGAY. Preliminary studies have shown that commercial heat wraps (such as the product ThermaCare) are more effective in relieving muscle pain than over-the-counter medication.*

- **Acupuncture:** *Several studies have suggested that pain from musculoskeletal conditions can be successfully treated by acupuncture. Many people have reported that it offers them significant pain relief without drugs, or has been an effective complement to their subscription drug therapy. As an acupuncturist, I can say that a large percentage of my patients respond well to this ancient pain-relief practice.*

- **Osteopathy:** *Osteopathy is a system of therapy that places an emphasis on the musculoskeletal system. FM patients may* *receive a full course of body manipulation therapies as part of a comprehensive treatment plan.*

- **Myofascial Release:** *The myofascial (from fascia, meaning tissue) release technique is utilized specifically to relieve tightness and restricted movement of the body's connective tissue. When correctly done it can help lengthen connective tissue and reduce its pull on the skeletal system. Some people report that this offers them long-term relief.*

- **Trigger Point Therapy:** *This technique was designed to break up the "trigger points" related to myofascial syndrome. A therapist who practices TPT will provide sustained pressure to help break up and relieve trigger point stress and pain. Use of a TENS device such as Dr. Ho's Muscle Massage System on trigger points can also be quite effective in releasing them, and with less discomfort for some than standard TP therapy.*

- **Craniosacral Therapy:** *This manual therapy was designed to help relieve bodily stress through applied gentle pressure to the back of the head (cranium) at the line of the ear. This treatment involves a commercially available product called the Still Point Inducer, but one can be fabricated at home by arranging two tennis balls inside a sock. A therapist practicing this therapy may be available near you, or you may be able to find more information online.*

- **Occupational Therapy:** *Specifically designed for people whose jobs contribute to their FM symptoms (repetitive motion tasks and/or a non-ergonomic working environment, for example), an occupational therapist can help by suggesting and implementing improvements in the workplace to provide relief and help prevent future problems.*

- **Relaxation Therapy:** *Naturally anyone dealing with the stress of FM (along with the stressors of everyday life) needs to be attentive to the effects stress can take on one's life. FM's symptoms can be induced and worsened by stress, so it is important to incorporate relaxation therapy as part of a permanent lifestyle commitment. There are many to choose from — yoga, meditation, guided imagery, biofeedback, breathing therapy, gentle martial arts like Tai Chi, even sensory deprivation (where you lie still in a tank filled with water) — and have all shown to offer relief from stress. Check your local bookseller on online resource for books or audio tapes on the therapies that most interest you and make sure you find something you can live with for the long term.*

- **Cognitive Therapy:** *Negative thinking can have damaging effects on anyone's well-being. It is vitally important to maintain a positive attitude about yourself and your health, even during times when you are suffering symptoms. Being diagnosed with FM can be a stressful experience and can cause some people to feel betrayed, angry or depressed. Any of these reactions is normal and understandable, but not to be ignored. If your feelings of anger or depression do not go away by a few weeks after your original diagnosis, or if you are feeling helpless, guilty or as though you have been victimized by bad luck or by your body, it will help you immensely over the long run to rid yourself of those feelings. FM is a disorder that affects millions of people worldwide. It is not your fault that you have it. You did nothing to invite it; it is not a punishment. Most people have situations occur in life that take them by surprise and cause them to alter some aspect of their lifestyle. What is important to remember is that you do have some control over your body and your symptoms, and that you have absolute control over your lifestyle. Most importantly, FM does not* *define who you are – you are still the same wonderful person you were before you were diagnosed.*

If you find yourself given to long bouts of negative thinking, cognitive/behavioural therapy (support groups, classes, audio- and videotapes, and individual counselling) can be of tremendous benefit to get you back to feeling like yourself again.

Keeping a Positive Attitude

It can be difficult to stay positive when you wake up stiff and sore: you're forced to call in sick to work, your spouse mutters under his or her breath when you say you're too tired to go out *again*, your kids are demanding time and energy you just don't have, and you have a long list of things that have to get done but you just don't feel up to tackling them. This can be a typical day for an FM sufferer – trying to stay upbeat can be a real challenge.

But happiness, like anything else in life, can take practice. Few of us, even those who don't have a physical condition that demands our attention, have a complete mastery of happiness. It can take work to be happy, as odd as that sounds. Some people manage to grasp the concept of happiness quite well: they deal wonderfully with adversity and always look ahead with great optimism. They're the people we know who are usually fun to be around and whose lives seem close to perfect. The truth is, they face most of the same problems that bother the rest of us – they just do it with a better attitude, and that makes all their bad times easier to overcome and their good times easier to enjoy.

You don't have to have been born this type of person, but you can *practice* being positive, just like you'd practice a musical instrument or a dance step. How do you practice being happy? By constantly reminding yourself of some dos and don'ts:

DO:

- *Make having fun a priority, just as you would prioritize a job or your family. Set aside at least thirty minutes every day to do something you want to do. Read, take a walk, call a friend, sit outside in your garden, paint; take regular pleasure breaks, alone or with positive people who make you feel good. Then, once a week, do something bigger that you love, like meeting friends for lunch or a movie or to go sailing. If you can find something wonderful to do with your family, so much the better. Make these events easy to do and inexpensive so that finances won't keep you from enjoying yourself.*

- *Have hobbies that provide enjoyment, escape and a sense of fulfillment. The hobby can be anything: bowling, sketching, singing, writing, whatever you wish. Don't limit yourself to something you're good at. If you want to take up the trombone, do it (even if you have to play it in the garage). You don't have to be good — you just have to have fun.*

- *Practice bravery. A lot of FM patients hesitate to make big plans like trips for fear that their symptoms will force them to cancel. What often happens is that the fear and anxiety of waking up in terrible pain on the day you're supposed to go hiking or get on a plane actually invites the pain by tensing your muscles. Start small, but make plans and keep them. Then as you get more comfortable with your capabilities, make bigger plans. Eventually, you will learn your true limits instead of your imagined ones and you will probably be pleasantly surprised.*

- *Exercise. Do it every day, whether you want to or not, for at least twenty minutes. Don't overdo it – you have nothing to prove to anyone. Your motives should be to stay healthy and flexible and feel better, not to run a marathon (unless you want to make it a long-term goal). In the meantime, be kind to yourself, but don't let your pain keep you down.*

- *Ask for support when you need it. Don't think that those around you can't help or that you have no right to ask. If your spouse or best friend broke his or her leg, you'd be there in a second to help fix dinner, do dishes or laundry, or just to provide a good ear. It's okay if your condition is more permanent than a broken leg – this is a physical ailment that you didn't ask for and which can cause problems, and those who care about you can provide help when the situation demands it. So ask!*

DON'T:

- *Let negative thoughts take over. If you find yourself blaming or being angry with yourself because of your FM, force yourself to stop in your tracks. It isn't your fault, nor is it anyone else's. It's just a fact. Not a very pleasant fact, for sure, but look at your condition realistically. When you begin to feel angry at yourself or at the world, tell yourself, "I'm having a bad moment and it will pass. This moment is not my life and it does not define who I am. I'll wait for this bad moment to fade and when it does, I'll feel like myself again."*

- *Let people give you unwanted advice. It seems that everyone you meet knows someone who knows someone who can cure your FM. Listen if you believe the person deserves an open mind, but if you don't believe that their advice will be helpful (or if they're being pushy), just thank them for their concern and change the subject. Or even politely leave their company if they cause you stress. It isn't your responsibility to listen just because someone feels like talking.*

- *Waste valuable moments. If you wake up feeling great, treat it like a "day off" and fit as much pleasure into it as you can. If you have a roster of unpleasant tasks that you need to deal with, then select only those that absolutely must get done and leave the others for another day. Sometimes good health demands putting yourself first and things of lesser importance on a back burner.*

- *A good attitude will not only decrease your emotional tension, but your physical tension as well. Think of being positive as therapy just like exercise: you need it to feel and be your best.*

In Summary

Regular rest and exercise, physical and emotional therapy, massage, relaxation therapy, healthy eating habits and the appropriate use of the right medications can help control the symptoms of fibromyalgia. Some people who manage their **FM** judiciously have minimal symptoms for the rest of their lives. Just take care of yourself, ask for help when you need it and don't let irrational negative thoughts take over, and there's no reason that **FM** should stop you from living a full and happy life.

Notes:

Treatment and Prevention

This is likely the chapter that you've been most anxious to read, and I will do my best to make sure your patience is rewarded.

The treatment and prevention of the pain syndromes associated with cervical spine muscle tension and spasm share some things in common, as well as other characteristics that are specific to particular disorders. So let's first discuss some universal truths about health and pain treatment and prevention – these are guidelines that will apply to everyone, so I encourage you to read them, no matter what symptoms you have or disorder(s) you suffer. In the next section you can refer to additional information that highlights your particular problem. By the end of the chapter you should have a complete idea of how to apply at-home treatment for your pain as well as how to achieve and maintain good overall health.

First, let's revisit the platform established in chapter 1 that describes the correct environment for good health through the *four pillars of health*: the physical pillar, the neuro-energetic pillar, the chemical pillar and the psycho-emotional pillar. Each of these must perform adequately in order to establish and maintain your physical condition.

How Can I Support My Physical Pillar?

If you recall from chapter 1, the physical pillar deals with your basic anatomy – your skeletal and muscular system. It addresses how well your spine is aligned, how fully your joints function and how strong and flexible your muscles are.

Some of the factors that can jeopardize the physical pillar are our own faults – we may be guilty of long periods of inactivity or ignore injuries, allowing them to become worse due to overuse or simple disregard. But many are not our fault, simply bad luck. Not one of us was born perfect; we may have congenitally flat feet, a curved spine or suffer muscular dysfunction that we neither invited nor caused. Or we may have had an accident at some point in our lives that caused us to suffer permanent or ongoing damage. If you were born with or acquired a disease or spine malformation or another problem that interferes with your physical pillar of health, it isn't the end of the world. It merely offers you a greater challenge. And much can be done to correct disorders associated with the flaws in one's anatomy.

Because I am a chiropractor, you may be inclined to conclude that I will suggest that every person who suffers a spinal malformation or injury or a muscular dysfunction should *visit* a chiropractor. The truth is that no two people are the same and not everyone will respond to the same corrective treatment. Also true is that not all chiropractors are the same – quite honestly, some are better than others. You or someone you know may have had a bad experience with chiropractic treatment. Naturally it would be impossible for me to say if that bad experience was caused by your individual problem's lack of response to appropriate treatment, or because your chiropractic treatment was inappropriate or poorly administered. But if you've given such treatment a fair try and received little or no relief (or found that your symptoms worsened), certainly don't continue with it.

In favour of chiropractic care, I have to say that I've treated thousands of people and the majority have responded well to it for a variety of reasons. For one, chiropractors do not dispense pain medications and are therefore far more compelled to treat conditions at their source than most MDS, who can easily write a prescription for pain meds and move along to the next patient. Another reason is that for many patients chiropractic attention is the "last line of defense" against pain – traditional care has failed and they've become desperate enough to try "unconventional" therapies. And along with the standard chiropractic treatment, which utilizes spinal manipulation and movement to correct certain misalignments and muscle constriction, chiropractors are usually far more open to other forms of holistic treatment, including massage therapy, TENS therapy, stretching exercises such as yoga and emotional support systems like meditation and biofeedback. This wider array of treatment options gives patients far more to work with and greater control over their therapy, since some curatives may work well for some and not for others. Being offered the limited options that most MDS provide seldom accounts for anyone's individuality and therefore may not come close to giving every patient the full course of pain remedies he or she may need to find relief.

Supporting the physical pillar of your health will be more complicated for some than for others. If you were born with a condition of the spine such as scoliosis, for example, you may require ongoing care to help relieve the pressure on your body. Addressing every specific spinal maladaptation would be a book in and of itself and more than I can accurately address here. But I can provide common-sense suggestions that apply to all people, whether they are in perfect health or not. My philosophy consists of common-sense approaches to health, vitality, longevity and pain reduction.

You have a great influence over your skeletal and muscular health, even if you don't find yourself being aware of either. As for your skeletal alignment, the biggest enemy your spine may suffer won't always be a car accident or even a condition like scoliosis, but your posture.

A Brief Discussion on Posture

In my experience most people have at least some posture problems. If you don't think this generalization applies to you, try the following: pretend that a string is attached to the top of your head and goes straight up toward the ceiling. This is correct head and neck posture and it is what you should assume whenever you drive, talk on the phone, watch TV, type, etc. It is very likely that many of you don't adopt this posture most of the time, and I urge you to work on making a habit of it. This posture allows the occipital bone, the one at the lower rear part of your skull, to sit in alignment with the *atlas,* the thin "platform" just beneath it and directly above the top of the cervical spine. It allows the head to relieve itself of gravity's pull, takes weight off the neck muscles and helps to maintain your upper spine's cervical curve.

Far too many X-rays that I view of patients' cervical spines reveal upper vertebrae that are straightened, kinked or pushed forward. This malformation of the spine occurs over time and is due almost exclusively to a lifetime of bad head positioning. Your head should not spend most of its time *angled forward,* as if it is leading your body. Rather, think of the column of your neck as a balancing point for the weight of your head. When you sit at a table or desk, the mission should be to position whatever you're doing to allow your head to sit atop the atlas without angling forward for long periods. How are you sitting while reading this book? Is your head dipped to read the print instead of the book being positioned to keep your head level on your neck? If so, is this a habit? If your answer is yes, you will need to practice changing how you do some common activities, including reading, working, watching TV and sleeping.

Let's take work for example. You should always sit upright while typing; if you find yourself tilting your head forward of your chest then your monitor is too far away or your default font is too small or, if your wear glasses, your prescription needs adjusting. Work that demands your head to be angled forward, such as assembly work of any kind, may be harder to manipulate. But being conscious of your posture will allow you to remember to take frequent breaks and move your head and neck to limit the pressure on your cervical spine and the muscles that support it.

Phones present another unique problem, one that can be more serious than many of us may understand. Too many people suffer from neck-related problems due to incorrect use of the telephone. Problems range from simple muscle tension to what is known as a mini-stroke, an alarming condition in which a person temporarily loses control of speech, some or all vision and may experience hearing impairment. This is not an affliction of the aged, but can happen among younger people, as was recently documented in a case involving a forty-three-year-old psychiatrist who favoured cradling the telephone between his left ear and shoulder so that he could take notes during conversations with patients. This simple ongoing act of bad posture caused a bony structure called the *styloid process*, a bone that runs along either side of the skull behind the jaw, to rupture his carotid artery, a major vessel that supplies the brain. Although his stroke symptoms subsided within a few hours, they served as a frightening wake-up call for him to correct what had become a bad habit. If you talk on the phone regularly, I suggest investing in a headset or speakerphone system.

If you don't speak on the phone often enough to warrant such devices, at least be certain not to cradle the phone between your neck and shoulder and to switch ears every few minutes of conversation. During long calls, take a few seconds to move your head side to side to keep your synovial juices flowing.

With regard to walking, running and other standing activities, the same is true – your head should not lead your body, but should sit on top of it and allow its weight to be supported. The entire posterior side of your body, from the back of your head to the base of your spine where it meets your buttocks, is shored up by "slow-twitch" muscles that do well with long-term activities – such as supporting your body's weight, balance and alignment – but are also very prone to muscular tension. The muscular tension in turn decreases the oxygen these muscles receive, increasing the pain and the chance of injury from even minor trauma. Once a certain level of tension has persisted for a long enough period, these muscles can become trained to stay tense, a condition known as segmental facilitation, causing ongoing agony even after the period of injury or stress has passed.

Part of preventing segmental facilitation is to limit the stress these muscles must bear day to day – bad posture places too much pressure on one muscle or a set of muscles and from there the problems begin. For example, angling your head forward for long periods places undo stress on the trapezius muscles that support your cervical spine. And since the trapezius also runs down into your upper back and across to your shoulders, the tension spreads rapidly across your upper body, where it can affect other muscles until whole regions ache as if they're on fire.

Ultimately there is a proper posture for almost all activities in life and being aware of and utilizing the tools that encourage proper posture is a system called *ergonomics*.

How Does Ergonomics Work?

Ergonomics focuses on the principle of minimizing stress on the body's muscles and joints. It has evolved in recent years from the increase of modern injuries like repetitive stress disorders and chronic muscle tension. The concept of ergonomics sprang from common complaints, such as large numbers of computer workers being afflicted with carpal tunnel syndrome, and quickly spread into all areas of life such as driving and sleeping. Ergonomics is really nothing more than an adjustment – either in the way a desk sits in relationship to your body or how you sit in an ordinary chair – that supports proper body alignment. And it's a concept that cannot be limited only to the workplace, but applied to all aspects of your life.

Under the laws of physics and body mechanics, the skeletal system and its supporting muscles function like a machine. The core of the skeletal framework is the spine, which in its natural posture resembles a gentle *S* when being viewed from the side. From behind, the spine should be straight and the top of the pelvic bone should be level. The significance of this neutral spinal posture is that it must be maintained in order to minimize the amount of stress on the muscles and joints throughout the body. Keep this in mind while you read and practice the information I share with you in this chapter. In fact, keep it in mind *whenever* engaged in any activity, even the most mundane such as washing dishes. This will seem cumbersome at first, but once it becomes habit you won't have to think about it at all; it will become your new and improved version of "normal" and once your body adapts to it, it will become comfortable.

Think of how you relax, whether reclining in the tub or watching TV or whatever you do to forget about the stress of the day. Is your head angled on pillows that crank your spine into a forward arc? Lying on your back with a big fat pillow under your head so you can view a TV screen may seem like the ultimate relaxation technique, but you will need to be aware every minute of the day now about your head and its relative position to your body. This is not a good posture to relax in, because it can easily cause subtle neck strain that will become silently and progressively worse until it generates its own pain situation or at very least sets you up to be vulnerable to injury. I can hear some of you groaning at the idea of giving up this cherished posture, but it is like any bad habit – once you get past it, you won't miss it.

So how are you supposed to relax and watch TV without irritating your neck? If I told you that most North Americans watch too much TV, it wouldn't surprise you. If I suggested that you limit your TV viewing to a few hours a week, some of you would toss this book into the trash before you reached the end of the paragraph. So, in the interests of keeping as friends those among you who love television, just let me suggest some common-sense tips that will help you to stay loose and maybe even increase your enjoyment of our continent's favourite pastime:

- *Don't watch TV with your head propped forward or with the screen angled so that you have to turn your head to view it. A rolled-up towel behind your neck is often the best support you can get, so try out different towel sizes until you feel your head being supported in an upright position – neither pushed forward nor angled back. And make sure you move your head gently from side to side ten times every half an hour.*

- *Don't sit for more than thirty minutes at a time. At least every thirty minutes get up and move around: walk to the bathroom or to get a drink of water (don't use the opportunity to fill up your snack tray – it's one of the reasons that TV viewing is associated with an increase in North Americans' average weight over the past fifty years). Take a cue from your cat: the first thing a cat does after lying around for awhile is stretch out his back – a nice, long stretch that feels good and gets him ready to walk around. Gently stretch all areas of your spine, slowly and easily. Never force a stretch or overstretch, especially when your muscles are cold. Make this a habit and you'll be amazed at the long-term benefits.*

- *Don't let TV keep you away from regular exercise or from social activities. If you limit your TV viewing to only those shows you really want to see, you'll enjoy it more and watch it less.*

Sitting at Work

The best advice I can give on sitting is that you should try not to do it too much and if possible, not more than thirty minutes at a time. Select a chair that fits your body shape and size. The seat pan should be short enough that you can sit all the way to the back of the chair, but don't use this as an excuse to lean against the backrest while you're working. The backrest of a work chair is there to allow you to take breaks, but should be used only in a limited fashion – your back should be upright and away from the backrest during the lion's share of your seated activities, such as typing or writing. One exception, of course, is driving. Truthfully, a proper work break involves getting up rather than leaning back, but leaning back can be a nice change for a moment or two during longer periods of sitting.

The height from the floor should be adjustable so that your feet can rest flat on the ground. Using a solid and stable-angled footrest can help reduce the pressure on your back.

The backrest should be supportive but any work chair you use for long periods should not have a headrest such as so-called "executive" chairs have, since this places your head too far back off the atlas – the back panel should come up no higher than your shoulders. If your work chair has such a headrest, limit its use to only a moment or two every so often, and resist using it while on the phone for long periods. Having an adjustable armrest is also helpful in reducing the amount of stress on your neck and shoulders, and it can aid in reducing carpal tunnel and tennis elbow injuries. When sitting, aim your buttocks to the back corner of the seat to help prevent slouching. If you find your work chair uncomfortable and your employer resists replacing it, it may be worth your while to invest in one you like and bring it to work.

Setting Up Your Computer Workstation

This topic can be very extensive, so I will provide you with some basic guidelines to get you started. Much of the remainder, once you get accustomed to maintaining neutral spinal posture, is common sense.

Always organize your work desk according to your task. The basic equipment I will take into account here will be the keyboard, the mouse and mouse pad, the monitor, the telephone and the writing surface. The piece of equipment that you use the most throughout the day is what should be placed directly in front of you. For example, if you spend 80 percent of your work time writing by hand, then your writing surface should be directly in front of you and the monitor and keyboard should be positioned to the side.

If you tend to work at the computer most of the time, place the monitor and keyboard directly in front of you. I prefer adjusting the height of the monitor so that the centre of the screen is level to the tip of my nose – this will help to maintain neutral posture of the neck and upper back. The keyboard should be positioned so that while you type your bent arms form a ninety-degree angle. Using wrist supports, which are available in great variety at many stores, should enhance this relief, though be sure to pick the kind that works most effectively for you – it's easy to test them because the benefits should be felt immediately.

When utilizing the mouse or keyboard, try to maintain a neutral alignment of the wrists (not bent but straight) and "float" your fingers and hands over the keyboard as you type. Your elbows should sit comfortably near your sides, so that your bent arms create a ninety-degree angle. Use wrist pads and arm rests only to take frequent breaks – don't rest your palms or forearms while typing. If you're reading while keying in, it is best to have the information on a stand beside the monitor in an upright position. Also, try to alternate the hard copy from the left to right side to prevent neck strain caused by looking too long in one direction. If you find yourself leaning forward to read your monitor, it may be too far away or your default font size may be set too small. Adjust both until you can clearly see the information on your screen without hunching or leaning forward.

When using a telephone, use a headset or speakerphone whenever possible to reduce the strain on your neck and shoulder muscles. If you don't have a headset, always hold the phone receiver with your hand while keeping your neck and shoulders in a neutral posture. If it's a long call, switch ears every few minutes. *Do not* squeeze the phone between your neck and shoulder. If you do, neck strain will erupt within only a few minutes.

Position manuals, catalogues and other books on your shelves according to their weight and frequency of use. The heaviest manuals that you use most often should be placed the closest to you, within easy reach. Your workstation is like the cockpit of an airplane: organize it to fit your needs and you will function most effectively and feel better while doing it.

Even when set up most efficiently, sitting and working at your desk for long hours will still cause major repetitive stress to the body. Regular neck, shoulder, forearm and wrist massage, either from a friend or therapist or by using a TENS device such as *Dr. Ho's Muscle Massage System*, and the special exercises I detail in this book will relieve and remedy the stress of wear and tear. Try to employ both massage and exercise on a regular (preferably daily) basis. I suggest getting up from your chair every half-hour to take a few minutes to perform the exercises for your neck, upper back, lower back and wrists. Over time, you'll be glad that you did.

Other Tips to Help Prevent Work-Related Injuries

- *Prepare for your workday. If you work at a job, arrive five to ten minutes early and take a brisk walk around the area, just enough to get your heart rate up. It will loosen you up after your commute and warm up your muscles to make them less prone to injury during the day. It's simple, easy and requires nothing more than a few minutes. Plus, without even noticing it, it adds one hundred to two hundred extra minutes of activity to your month. Over the course of the year, without even trying you'll burn enough extra calories to drop five to ten pounds, even more if you are presently overweight.*

- *Take more breaks. By "breaks" I don't mean talking on the phone or some other activity that might add to your neck's tension, but actually give your body a break. Clearly you probably can't leave your desk every half an hour to walk around the lobby, but you can stand up from your chair and stretch for thirty to sixty seconds.*

When I say stretch I don't mean touching your toes or another advanced stretch that should be done when the body is warm, but gentle "feel good" stretches. Wiggle your fingers, shake your hands, gently stretch your back, move and massage your neck. It takes only a few seconds and it can prevent years of stiffness and suffering.

- *Drink more water. One of the great ways to take regular breaks is by doing something most of us need to do more often anyway: drink water. Drink a four-ounce glass of water every half-hour. Yes, you'll have to go to the bathroom more often – that's the point. It forces you to get up regularly without thinking about it, it gets you to walk around, both to eliminate and to get a refill of water. By the end of the day, you'll have had 64 oz. of water, which is the recommended amount for the average person for the entire day. You'll be better hydrated and you'll feel better, too. And then you can limit your consumption in the hours close to bedtime, to help prevent waking in the night with a full bladder.*

Sitting at Home and During Rest

Sit upright in a chair or other type of seating that supports your whole spine, from your lower back to your upper back, but let your head balance itself as much as possible. Avoid propping your head on fat pillows or too many pillows that might force your head forward of your neck. Frequent use of headrests can force your head too far back and off its centre balance and can lead to serious problems over the long term, such as segmental facilitation, disc herniation and cervical spondylitis. If you want to rest your head against something, a rolled-up towel or neck roll can provide good support and keep your head and neck in better alignment than will a headrest.

Sitting in Your Car

It is important to note that the headrest in your car is really there to help prevent whiplash and should be considered an important preventive measure, *not* a place to rest your head while driving. Make sure to keep your head balanced levelly on top of your neck while you drive and rest your head, if you want, only when stopped at a light. You should also take this time to move your fingers and arms if you've been holding the steering wheel for more than a few minutes. Cradling a cellphone while driving is not only a good recipe for an accident, it can cause great neck strain. If you must talk while driving, I highly recommend a telephone headset, which will not only take stress off your neck but also may very well keep you from suffering a car accident. Remember that even the classic "fender-bender" serves as a very effective "onset event" for neck and spinal problems.

As often as possible and *at least* every hour, get out of your car and gently stretch your spine, move your legs and rotate your head from side to side twenty times or more to keep your cervical joints mobile and lubricated.

Sleeping Posture

Sleeping is another issue. If you sleep consistently on your back (probably the best sleeping posture for your spine), your pillow should be low profile, that is, not high enough to force your head forward. You should also place a pillow beneath your knees so that your lumbar spine is allowed to naturally flatten and be supported by your mattress. Most people sleep on their sides, however, and trying to train yourself to sleep on your back can be difficult, or even impossible if you're prone to a lot of movement during sleep. But sleeping on your side is fine provided you get into a few habits.

Your pillow should provide good support – not so low that your head dips toward your mattress and not so high that your head angles up toward the ceiling. For this reason, never use more than one pillow. The best pillows are malleable, so that they conform around your neck and face and don't push against them, but rather provide comfortable support. Ergonomic pillows made of a slow-contracting polyurethane foam are sometimes shaped to support the neck and some people find them comfortable, but others find them awkward. They have even been known to aggravate underlying neck problems, so use them only if they feel good and make you sleep better. Pillows made of polyurethane typically produce a peculiar chemical smell that can be slow to go away. If you're highly sensitive to smells (as are many people, particularly those who get migraines or suffer from fibromyalgia) and you want to try out a urethane-based pillow, I suggest that you unwrap it as soon as you get it home and before you use it place it in a well-ventilated area for a few days or even weeks, until the smell goes away. And again, if you don't find the pillow comfortable, don't use it at all.

Whatever pillow you use, make sure you position your head so that your neck is supported by the gentle loft of the pillow and that your head is in line with your spine. If you have trouble determining your alignment, ask someone to look at your spine when you're in your usual sleeping position and tell you if it looks straight. Place your head so that your chin is not tilted toward your chest, but solidly against the pillow's surface. To further encourage proper spinal alignment, sleep with a medium-loft pillow between your knees, to keep your hips from forcing your lumbar spine to one side. Switch sides often to make sure your body doesn't adapt to being positioned only one way. If you sleep solidly through the night without moving, it will be especially important to keep track of which side you slept on the night before and sleep on the other the next night.

If you sleep on your belly, then you've got some adjusting to do. You should never sleep on your belly, because it forces the entire length of your spine into improper alignment, and will cause neck and back pain. To convert yourself to being a back sleeper, try lying comfortably on your back with a pillow beneath your knees while hugging a pillow against your chest. After a few days of training, you might be able to sleep on your back more easily.

As for your mattress, a firm one will usually provide better support than a soft or mushy one. If your mattress is getting old, saggy or has permanent body depressions in it, it's time for a new one. What you select should be based upon comfort, not price. Some incredibly expensive mattresses may not provide enough support or may be uncomfortable. Don't buy a mattress that feels uncomfortable just because the label says it's "ergonomic" or is good for your back. Lie on it for as long as possible (possibly until the store manager is about ready to ask you to leave!) and see how it feels. If you feel well-supported by a mattress that feels comfortable, it's likely a good choice.

Standing

Bending over even slightly and holding yourself in that position for any period of time can cause stress on your neck, shoulders and lower back muscles. Imagine you have a heavy bowling ball attached to the end of a stick. If the stick is balanced in an upright position, it'll take minimal effort to hold it up. However, if you hold it in a slightly tilted position, this will greatly increase the amount of required effort. Your body works the same way: leaning forward has the same stressful effect on the postural muscles along the spine.

Performing Chores

- **Vacuuming, Sweeping and Mopping**

Vacuuming, sweeping and mopping can be straining to your back muscles. To minimize the stress on them, keep your strokes very short so that you don't have to lean over. Furthermore, bend your knees to decrease the strain on the lower back. Maintain the neutral spinal posture as much as possible.

- **Cleaning the Bathtub**

Cleaning the bathtub can be so harmful to your back that there really isn't a proper way of doing it. My best advice is simply don't do it if you have a bad back; try to find someone with a strong back to do it for you. If you have to do it (even if you're a person with a strong back), I suggest getting right inside the tub, bending down on both knees and supporting the weight of the body with one arm. Use the other arm to do the cleaning. Absolutely do not stand outside the tub and lean over it to clean, as this is extremely incapacitating to the lower back muscles.

- **Making the Bed**

Never try to lean over for any prolonged period of time, no matter what you're doing. Always remember to maintain the neutral spinal posture. When reaching down to make the bed, for example, place your legs apart and stand with both heels flat on the ground. Bend the knees, not the back, to squat down low enough to reach the bed. If you have to reach across the mattress, rest one knee on the bed to support your lower back.

- **Carrying Bags**

Carrying bags of groceries or school books, and especially carrying a fully loaded handbag, can cause strain to your neck, shoulders and lower back muscles. Try to carry an equal amount of weight in each hand or arm, and try to use bags with double straps in order to balance the load. Carrying a bag or backpack on one shoulder causes the entire spine to bend and spreads stress to the lower back, neck and shoulder regions. Instead, try carrying your bags under your arm — this is much less stressful on your muscles. Never carry very heavy objects with straight arms, as it can lead to rotator cuff injury.

- **Bending, Lifting and Twisting**

Even if you know how to lift properly and the typical loads you lift tend to be light, please pay close attention to the following details. It is so important to bend, lift and twist in a manner that will minimize the amount of stress on your muscular and skeletal system.

1. *Square up, get close to your load and stand with your feet shoulder-width apart. Keep your heels flat on the ground at all times.*
2. *To bend down, bend your knees and hips. Do not bend the lower back.*
3. *Grab the load and bring it close to your body. Tighten up the abdominal muscles by exhaling.*
4. *While keeping your neutral spinal posture, lift up using your legs and buttocks.*
5. *To move your load to the side, do not twist your back, but always use your feet to reposition yourself so that your body is square to the location of unloading.*
6. *To unload, bend your knees and let your thighs bear the weight. Again, do not bend your lower back.*
7. *With awkward and/or heavy objects, always get some help. No matter what, always take the time to do what is right for your body.*

- **Gardening**

  When gardening, one tends to bend over for a substantial period of time. Using a kneepad or a small box to sit on will minimize the strain on your back and neck. Do not stay in one position for too long because it can cause your neck and back muscles to tighten up. Instead, try rotating from activity to activity rather than spending a long time doing one and then a long time doing the next. Or, if you're performing the same task for an extended duration of time, at least take rests and approach the job from different positions — while maintaining the neutral spinal posture as well as possible.

- **Shoveling**

  When shoveling, lift the full shovel using your legs to support the weight, turn with your feet rather than your trunk, and then use both your arms and your legs to propel the load. As with any situation in which you're holding something heavy and moving it to another location, bear the load with your thighs and don't twist your trunk at any time — doing so could invite anything from a pulled muscle to a herniated disc. Place any heavy load on your legs, always control what you carry or move, and never jerk, twist or make an uncontrolled or extreme movement. Better to shovel fifty light loads than twenty that are too heavy for the weaker parts of your body — such as your neck or lower back — to bear.

- **Putting Cargo In and Taking It Out of the Car Trunk**

  When moving heavy items in or out of the car trunk, rest one leg inside the trunk or against the bumper to transfer the weight from your lower back muscles to your legs. Bending over to lift heavy items is a classic way to invite lower back, shoulder and neck strain, so if the item is a challenge ask someone for help.

Life's Other Challenges

During episodes of pain or times of extreme stiffness, life's routines can represent major challenges. Because the spine's three sections, the cervical, the thoracic and the lumbar, are all part of the same structure – the spinal column – being kind to your cervical spine should involve looking at the spine as a whole. People in agony are often made almost immobile by it, or even after their injury subsides they can be left feeling fearful and vulnerable to a recurrence of their pain. So for many of us, simple tasks like getting into and out of bed can cause concern. Here are some ways to help eliminate the pain and fear involved in some of life's more mundane tasks:

- **Getting In and Out of Bed**

  Always consider the state that your body is in both when you get into bed after the end of a long day, and when you get out of bed after being immobile for hours, leaving your body sensitive to the most basic movements. There are six basic movements to properly get out of bed:

  1. *Turn on your side to face the closer edge of the bed.*
  2. *Let your legs hang over the side.*
  3. *Push up with the elbow and the supporting hand into a sitting position.*
  4. *Slide forward until both feet are on the ground.*
  5. *Lean forward to shift your weight and centre of gravity over your legs.*
  6. *Push yourself up with both arms.*

  To get in, take the same steps in reverse order.

- **Getting In and Out of the Car**

  If you have a lower back problem or neck strain that limits your ability to move your head, getting in and out of the car can be troublesome. Try doing it in two steps: first, stand facing away from the seat and lower your buttocks down gently so that you're sitting sideways on the seat. Then use your hands as leverage to assist your legs into the car. When leaving the car, get your legs out first and then pull yourself out of the seat, making sure your head doesn't bump against the door frame.

- **Getting On and Off the Toilet**

For most of us, getting on and off the potty is a relatively simple task. However, for those of us with back or spinal problems, it can be a challenge:

1. Try straddling the toilet.

2. Support your body weight with your arms on the tank and slowly lower yourself down.

3. To get off, use both your legs and arms to push yourself up.

Some people have no problem getting down on the toilet seat, but have a hard time lifting themselves back up because they're sitting so low. In this situation, try leaning as far forward as possible to put your centre of gravity over your knees, and then push up with both your arms and legs at the same time. Having fun yet?

Exercise and Stretching

Much of injury treatment and prevention has to do with establishing and maintaining the fluidity of the cervical muscles. If you have neck muscle stiffness or any related malady (and even if you don't but want to prevent them), you should begin implementing a series of simple exercises and stretches that will become as much a part of your daily routine as brushing your teeth. Always follow these stretching guidelines and even those of you who think you don't like to stretch will become converts:

- **Always warm up before stretching.** *The body's soft tissues (muscles, tendons and ligaments) are like taffy – when warm they stretch fine, when cold they resist being moved. A warm-up takes only five to ten minutes of gentle movement, such as walking around until you feel your body loosen up. In a pinch, you can also stretch after a hot shower or bath.*

- **Never stretch into pain.** *Done properly, stretching feels good. Stretch only into gentle resistance, or comfortable pressure. Stretching beyond your body's capabilities will not make you more flexible; in fact, it can lead to injury that will actually decrease your range of movement. Becoming flexible can take a long time for some people, but done daily and with commitment, you can train your muscles and soft tissues to relax and lengthen.*

- **Breathe deeply while you stretch.** *A common mistake people make is that they hold their breath during a stretch, which is never a good idea. Stretching enables your muscles to relax and receive greater blood flow (hence increased oxygen), so always take nice deep breaths during your whole routine. Once you get in the habit of breathing deeply, you can implement proper breathing for relaxation: breathe in deeply through your nose (this allows you to intake more air) and exhale slowly through your mouth. This is optimal breathing for stretching and relaxation, but some people find it confusing – if you do, just concentrate on breathing normally but deeply.*

- **Stretch before and after exercise.** *Before you undertake a specific exercise, such as jogging, weight training, playing golf or doing heavy lifting or even housework, do some gentle stretches to* *limber up. Then, just as importantly, stretch again after exercise to release lactic acid and the other chemicals that get trapped as muscles tighten up after stress. Your muscles will be warm after their labour and you can often make the most gains in flexibility after exercising.*

Since the topic of this book is maladies related to neck muscle tension, let's start with some simple exercises and stretches for the neck and then move on to some for the whole body.

Exercises and Stretches for the Neck

The following exercises will help strengthen the muscles in your neck and help to relieve existing neck pain and to prevent injury. Try them out and do them gently. If any are uncomfortable or increase your symptoms, don't do them. Everyone is different, so some stretches will work for some of you and won't for others. Do each exercise slowly and in a controlled fashion; never jerk or push your body beyond its comfort limits.

- **Simple Neck Stretch** – *gently let your head fall to the side, as if you were going to rest it on your shoulder. Do not push beyond your natural, comfortable limit. Hold for six seconds and then slowly do the other side. Repeat this five times on each side (ten total). As you become more flexible, you can apply very gentle pressure with your hand and increase the length of time you hold the stretch.*

- **Simple Neck Movement** – *turn your head from side to side as far as you can, but comfortably, ten times for each side (twenty total). Never jerk your neck or push it beyond its comfort zone.*

- **Shoulder Shrugs** – *this simple exercise feels good and helps to increase the fluidity of your shoulder and neck muscles. Sit or stand fully erect and pull your shoulders straight up toward the ceiling. Hold for five seconds, then slowly release. Begin with two sets of five repetitions and increase the number of sets as your body will allow. If you work at a job requiring forward handwork such as typing or assembly work, do these for every thirty minutes of time spent working.*

- **The Dorsal Glide** – *this movement stretches the trapezius muscles along the back of the neck. Start by sitting or standing perfectly erect. Tuck your chin straight back (as if you were giving yourself a double chin) and gently glide your head backward as far as you can until you are looking toward the ceiling. Glide back only as far as you feel comfortable. Hold for five seconds and then release. Begin with two sets of five repetitions and increase the number of sets when your body allows.*

- **Passive Neck Movement** – *lie on your back on a mat or firm mattress with your knees bent and your feet on the floor or mattress. Make a hammock of your hands by interlocking your fingers and place them behind your head so that your head and neck feel supported. Completely relax your neck and let your head be supported by your hands. Gently move your head from side to side (using your hands – your neck should remain relaxed) by moving to its maximum comfortable limit. Repeat the side-to-side movement twenty times. Do as many sets of twenty as your body finds comfortable.*

- **Shoulder Lifts** – *lie face down on a mat or the floor with your arms against your body. Keeping your lower body against the* *ground, slowly lift your head and shoulders off the floor as high as you can without pain. Hold for five seconds and then slowly relax. Begin with two sets of five and increase the number of sets as your body will allow.*

- **Shoulder Stretch** – *lift your right arm in front of your body and gently pull your right elbow toward your left shoulder. Don't overstretch – this stretch should feel good. Feel the stretch through your shoulder and adjust the level of your elbow until you feel the most comfortable pressure in your shoulder/rotator cuff area. Hold for thirty seconds and repeat on the other side. Do this stretch two times on each side (four times total). This is very helpful just before doing chores, lifting heavy objects and playing sports.*

Daily Stretches and Exercises for the Whole Body

Whether you love exercise or you hate it, it is absolutely essential to partake in daily basic exercise. Regular movement helps to restore and maintain joint motion and restrict muscle tension. Without it, it's very easy for muscles and joints to tighten up and form fibrous and/or scar tissue that will further limit movement, create pain and make you prone to injury. Such tissue will also lead to osteoarthritis and other problems that used to be found mainly in the elderly but are now found in increasing numbers among younger people.

When you don't use your muscles regularly they become weak, causing your posture to become altered because your muscles lack balance and don't pull equally on your skeleton. Basic movements of the neck and shoulder area will stretch out muscles and restore joint movement. The exercises I'm about to teach you will strengthen your neck and shoulder muscles and will help you maintain good posture.

When approaching exercise, it's important to take a "Goldilocks" approach to it – not too much, not too little, but something perfectly in between: "just right." What is too much? Anything that causes your body to experience injury or discomfort. Too little? Too little is perhaps a bit easier to define, because it is important to move your body every day and to engage in aerobic activity at least three to four times a week, from brisk walking to biking to running, depending on your fitness level. No one can decide for you what is "just right," because everyone is different, but often your body will let you know. Too much and too little exercise can produce the same symptoms: stiffness, aching muscles and fatigue – warning signs to adjust your activity level. Even people who are very fit can suffer neck tension and its associated problems – many of the people I treat are athletes who either sustained injury from an accident or who are simply prone to muscle stiffness for the same reasons that some people are tall and some are short. One element of good health, after all, is luck. But to the very significant degree that we can make ourselves healthier, we should feel compelled to do everything we can out of sheer self-respect.

So don't try to match the achievements of other people when you decide to implement exercise into your life, especially if this is a new habit for you. I can't tell you how many injuries I treat that arise because two people get together for the first time to go jogging or play sports – one is fitter than the other but they feel pushed by competition to match achievements. This often leads the less fit person to overdo it and become injured.

The following daily routine, therefore, is designed to benefit anyone, whether fit or not. Of course if anything I recommend in this book is uncomfortable for your body, don't do it. These are just good basic "beginner" moves that prepare you for your day and help you to loosen up and prevent injury. If you have been sedentary for a long time or have health concerns, take this list to your doctor before you begin so that he or she can make recommendations specific to you and your condition.

No matter what your age or fitness level, it's never too late to try to restore your body's maximum range of motion. Easy passive movement and posture awareness exercises, not necessarily an aerobics class, are all that's required. But you need to be diligent about doing exercise regularly: don't do it only when you're feeling stiff and in pain, but religiously every day. The more prone to stiffness you are, the more you will benefit by doing these three to four times a day: first thing in the morning, during your lunch break, when you get home and just before bed. After four weeks of such a routine, you will be amazed at how much better you feel and more fluidly you move.

The following exercises are designed to improve your spinal flexibility, your mobility and your strength. Be sure to start out nice and easy when embarking on a new exercise program: it's a good idea to start with ten repetitions per exercise before gradually increasing to twenty, thirty, or even one hundred reps depending on your comfort level. The application of a **TENS** device, such as *Dr. Ho's Muscle Massage System,* will help ease tension in the muscles before and after these and other exercises.

Dr. Ho's Easy Daily Exercise Routine

1. *Start out by loosening up. Do an exercise I call "the twist": let your arms and shoulders go limp. Now begin by gently swinging your arms from side to side. Then start following your arm motion by moving your head in sync with your arms so that you can watch your hands swing to and fro. You'll find that you automatically involve your spine in the motion; this is great to loosen your spinal column.*

2. *Now stand tall and just move your neck. Look both ways, left and right, very gently. Repeat ten times on each side, then increase up to fifty or more as your body will allow.*

3. *Try some lateral flexion. Reach your hands above your head and lean gently to one side. Don't lean over farther than your comfort level. Some may find this stretch more comfortable if they leave their hands at their sides.*

4. *Do the "windmill" to loosen your shoulders: whip one arm down and let the momentum carry the weight of it back up, keeping the arm relaxed throughout. Do this ten times, first forward then backward. Follow with the other arm.*

5. *Stretch your lower back by placing your feet shoulder-width apart, bending your knees, and slowly bending over by curling one vertebra at a time until you can hold your ankles (or as far down as is comfortable – don't push farther than your ability). Hold gently and concentrate on letting your back muscles go nice and limp while your head dangles. Then slowly come back up, curling the spine back up one vertebra at a time, and reach for the sky.*

6. *Push-ups. For those of you who haven't done push-ups in a long*

time, you can do them horizontally: find yourself a solid table or counter and place your arms shoulder-width apart. You can move your legs away from the base according to the amount of tension you want to have. Do ten to thirty, adjusting to your own fitness level. Always do exercises at your own comfort level – it isn't necessary to push too hard.

7. *Here's a great stretch for your neck and chest muscles. Anchor your hand against the wall or door frame and turn your whole body with your feet. Also gently turn your neck. You know by now how important it is to stretch out these muscles around the neck area. If you work at repetitive tasks such as typing or assembly, do this at work several times a day.*

8. *Squatting. Stand with your feet shoulder-width apart, hold your arms out in front of you, keep your spine straight and then bend into a "sitting" position – not too deep, just until your thighs and calves form a ninety-degree angle. This is good for the gluteus maximus muscles, the hamstrings, the lumbar spine muscles and your whole supporting base. If this move makes you feel unstable, place a chair behind you so that if you lose your balance your posterior will meet the chair and not the floor.*

9. *Here's an exercise for your abs. Stand tall and hold your arms straight out in front of you. In a smooth, controlled motion, bring your right knee up to touch your right hand or arm. If you have trouble bringing your knees up this high you can adjust the level by lowering your arms.*

10. *A similar exercise for the oblique muscles (sometimes called your "love handles") is done by putting your arms out to the side at a ninety-degree angle, then bringing your knees, one at a time, up*

to the elbow on the same side. As far as frequency goes, you can do from ten to one hundred reps depending on your fitness level.

11. *Lower back, hip and spine stretch. Sit on the ground with your legs straight in front of you. Cross your right leg over your left and place your right foot flat on the ground. Place your left arm outside your right knee and push against the knee, then gently pull with your spine and turn your neck. You can support your body weight by putting the other hand on the ground. Don't push too hard. You should feel a nice gentle stretch happening in the lower back, hip area and in the neck.*

12. *Place your legs out and apart, then reach forward with one arm toward one leg. Grab your toe and bring the other arm across to hold your knee.*

13. *A variation of the last exercise involves bringing the opposite hand right around to grab the toe. You should always be concentrating on letting your muscles go loose, in this case the back muscles. Once you're a little more limber, you can bend forward to stretch the hamstring and lower back. When you're ready, you can increase the intensity by holding the ankle instead of the toe. Focus on letting go. You should be able to feel it right in the hamstring and lower back. Don't worry if you have a hard time with this. Just do it as well as you can every day and you'll become more flexible.*

14. *Sit on the floor and place the soles of your feet flat together so that your knees are sticking out to the sides. Hold your feet together with your hands and bend forward for about ten seconds. Don't you wish you were a teenager again? It gets harder and harder as you get older. This stretches the adductor*

muscles along the inner thigh.

15. *Now move onto your back. One of your most important muscles is the gluteus maximus (your buttocks). Place your arms out on the ground and push your body up in the air with your feet flat and your knees bent up. Hold for about ten seconds and feel your gluteus muscles contract, then come down slowly, relax.*

16. *Another stretch for the back: bend your knees with your backbone loose and pull them toward your chest with your arms. The small of your back should just come off the ground. This is great for your lower back and gluteus maximus. Muscles that are loose will have more power that those that are tight.*

17. *Another one for the same muscles is to lie flat on your back and bring one knee up and across toward the opposite shoulder. Hold it there with your hand for ten seconds. Repeat using the other knee.*

18. *Vertical push-ups. When you're strong enough from doing push-ups against the counter, you can do them on your knees. Keep your arms out a little wider than shoulder width, keep your spine straight and breathe out while you're exerting. The next step is being strong enough to do them on your toes. Keep your back straight throughout. It's good to change your speed for variation – fast and then slow. Push-ups will strengthen your neck and upper shoulder muscles, as well as improve your posture.*

Enjoy these easy exercises and remember that they should feel good. If you find yourself hating them, you may be pushing yourself too hard or too far, which won't accomplish anything. These should make you feel loose and relaxed when you finish and they often help people to sleep more deeply and wake up refreshed.

Keeping the Body Relaxed and Pain-Free With Massage

Massage is a technique used to manipulate muscles and cause deep tissue relaxation while promoting blood, lymphatic and nerve circulation. Massage can help to relieve pain, relax muscle spasms and promote faster healing. Although massage therapy is not intended to cure any life-threatening medical condition, it is widely used to manage daily stress and chronic pain.

To most people, a properly done massage feels wonderful. We get to let someone manipulate our stiff, tired and aching muscles while we simply relax. People who are well-off enough to afford a daily massage are lucky but a tiny minority. For the vast majority of us, massage is a special treat we may indulge in only rarely when we can justify the cost of pampering ourselves. What you may not know about massage, however, is that a proper massage is more than a pleasurable experience, it is actually beneficial to your health.

Appropriate massage techniques can relieve muscle tension and stiffness and stop spasm episodes. Regular massage reduces chronic pain, helps treat and prevent repetitive stress and overuse injuries, improves range of motion and helps push oxygen into tight muscles, enabling them to get rid of noxious pain chemicals and engage in damage repair. Massage improves blood circulation, bringing oxygen and nourishment to the body's soft tissues. Muscles are then able to relax, decreasing pain from all types of sources, from injury to arthritis to chronic stiffness, and reducing the chance of injury or reinjury.

Conditions that respond well to massage therapy are those

associated with tense muscles and poor circulation in the lymphatic, blood or nervous system. Many common painful conditions, such as migraine headaches, tension headaches, neck and shoulder pain, and upper and lower back pain, to name only a few, have been well-documented to respond favourably to massage therapy.

Many athletes utilize massage therapy to warm up and to treat specific sports-related muscle and tendon injuries such as those involving the shoulder rotator cuff, the elbow flexors and extensors, the hip flexors and the hamstring and quadriceps muscles of the thighs.

Massage encourages faster recovery of muscles that are overused from sports and repetitive strain injuries related to computers, musical instruments or physical labour. Everyone who uses their muscles repetitively at the same task should massage their necks, shoulders, forearms and wrists to treat and prevent repetitive strain injuries such as thoracic outlet and carpal tunnel syndrome. These conditions can cause neck pain, shoulder stiffness and pain in the forearms and hands sometimes accompanied by numbness or weakness. Massage therapy will provide immediate relief and prevent the condition from worsening.

Massage also allows your body's energy or "life force" to flow more effectively and efficiently through your body. This is something of foreign concept in Western culture, but it has been part of many Eastern cultures, particularly China's, for generations, and is a vital element in the implementation and teachings of acupuncture. And understanding your body's own energy balance brings us to the next pillar of health, your neuro-energetic pillar.

How Can I Support My Neuro-Energetic Pillar?

The neuro-energetic pillar is concerned with how well your nervous system flows and how efficiently your energy travels through your body. According to traditional Chinese medicine, any blockage of nerve and energy flow, known as *chi*, can cause pain and dysfunction in the body. Left untreated, this obstruction of one's *chi* can lead to chronic pain syndrome, premature degeneration, disease and even premature death.

Chinese medicine describes over three thousand pressure points that are mapped to identify each neuro-energy point in the body. One common and very effective preventative health practice is to regularly massage these pressure points to stimulate the nerves and promote the flow of energy. No, you don't need to know or need to massage all three thousand points – doing so would take all day and leave you exhausted! Luckily there are about a dozen key points that you can massage and stimulate regularly to maintain good health. Incidentally, many of these pressure points are located at the same areas where you very likely experience pain and tenderness when your body is under stress.

These key points include:

1. *The suboccipital area at the back of the neck just below the hairline.*
2. *The upper trapezius muscle belly.*
3. *The lateral side of the elbow.*
4. *The area on the hand between the thumb and index finger.*
5. *The mid-back just beside the shoulder blade.*
6. *The lower back at the level of the kidneys.*
7. *The lower back at the level of the pelvic crest.*
8. *The hip and centre of the buttock.*
9. *The area just behind the knee.*
10. *The area just below and to the right of the kneecap.*

11. *The area just above the inside of your ankle.*
12. *The area on the bottom of your feet.*

According to the teachings of acupuncture, your *chi* flows through these twelve key energy points. These energy pathways can be freed from blockages and beneficially stimulated by massage from your or someone else's hands, or through electrotherapy using a **TENS** device (which I'll discuss at length in the next section), to balance your energy and improve your body's operations – from your level of energy to your ability to have regular waste elimination.

Massage can aid your body's *chi* to move more smoothly and efficiently through its proper channels by eliminating the blocking factors (such as stress, tension and overexcited nerves) that can impede its progress.

Now that I've extolled the wonderful virtues of massage, you're probably thinking, "Well that's great, Dr. Ho, but as you stated yourself, most of us can't afford to get frequent massages." That's quite true. And not only is massage from a licensed therapist expensive, it's not very convenient for most of us. So what are you supposed to do? Do it at home.

The truth is that almost anyone can learn how to give a good, relaxing massage. Getting someone in your household or a good friend to perform one on you is another matter. But if you and your selected partner negotiate a trade system, you may find that regular massage is something you can plan into your life. I recommend that you and your partner massage each other on opposite days, provided your schedules will allow it: one person will get Monday, Wednesday and Friday, the other the following days, with one day off for both of you. If you require a daily massage, you may need to work out a system agreeable for both of you, such as alternating who goes first.

How Do You Give a Good Relaxation Massage?

A simple, general relaxation massage is easier to perform than most people think. All you need is a willing partner who will offer you feedback as you go so you can perfect your technique. People can get so accustomed to tension in their necks, backs and shoulders that they don't realize its presence until after a massage. A twenty-minute relaxation massage can make all the difference in releasing this tension and preventing its return. The important things to remember when performing massage are:

- *Some people like more pressure than others, but more pressure doesn't necessarily make for a better massage. Start gently, increase pressure slowly and only use as much as the person enjoys. Ask them to give you feedback on your technique as you go.*

- *In order to keep you from becoming tired as you massage, it's key to try to position your partner so that he or she is about the height of your waist (a massage table is of course ideal, but a table covered with a thick mat or folded blanket will also work. Lacking these, you can position your partner near the edge of a bed and sit directly next to him or her). You want to use your body weight as much as possible to apply pressure, rather than relying solely on your shoulders and hands, which will quickly become tired.*

- *Using oil will help your hands glide over the person's skin, limiting both the pressure you must apply and the irritation their skin may receive. Baby oil works well but, in a pinch, so will everyday vegetable oil. Massage oil has certain benefits (such as a nice smell and lasting lubrication), but it is often expensive.*

These points covered, let's get started. Your partner should lie face down and get comfortable. I find that placing a pillow beneath the front of the ankles takes some stress off the spine. Unless you have a massage table, it's likely that your subject will have to lie with their head twisted to one side, so I suggest that they switch their head position every so often so both sides of the neck will stretch evenly. Another solution is placing two large pillows underneath the chest (but not under the head), which will allow your subject's neck and head to fall forward into a neutral position. It's good to start out a massage with gentle palm pressure from the top to the bottom of the back – a general loosening technique to relax the joints between each vertebra.

From there, let's move to the neck. Apply gentle, firm, comfortable and rhythmic pressure – it should be like gently kneading dough. As you go, your partner will usually begin to loosen up and relax, allowing you to apply slightly more pressure. Ask him or her to let you know if they want more or less pressure. Both the subject and the masseuse (or the masseur, but for purposes of this text we'll use the more familiar "masseuse") should exhale slowly and deeply as the pressure is applied.

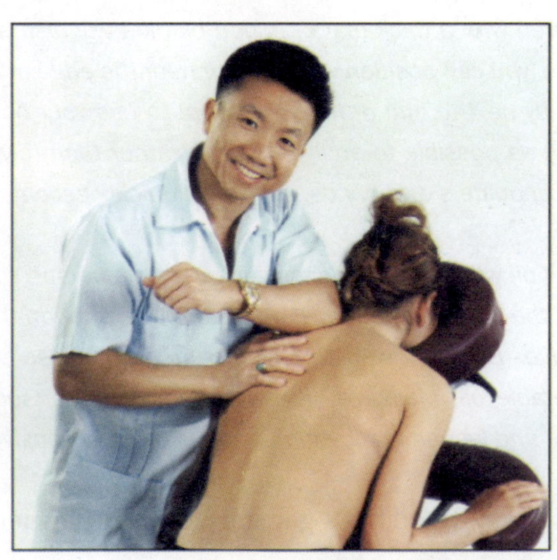

Now let's try another technique and apply direct steady thumb pressure along both sides of spine – the upper shoulder in particular holds a lot of pressure that needs to be released. Basic thumb pressure is one of the most effective procedures. Just use your body weight to press your thumbs against the muscles that support the spine, hold for a moment and then release, then inch your way down until you've covered the whole spine. To cover a wider area or to relieve pressure on your thumbs, you can use your elbow to apply pressure. Just remember to start gently because your elbow is capable of engaging more pressure than your thumb and lacks the thumb's sensitivity. Move up and down the sides of the spine using your own body weight. If you're standing, use your legs to transmit the weight instead of leaning over too much.

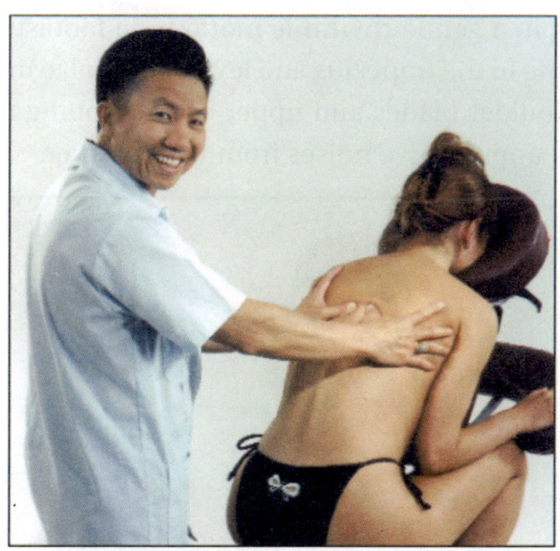

The muscle cross-fibre technique consists of pushing the thumbs toward each other all along spine. This is an excellent method to loosen up the many small muscles around the spine that can get restricted.

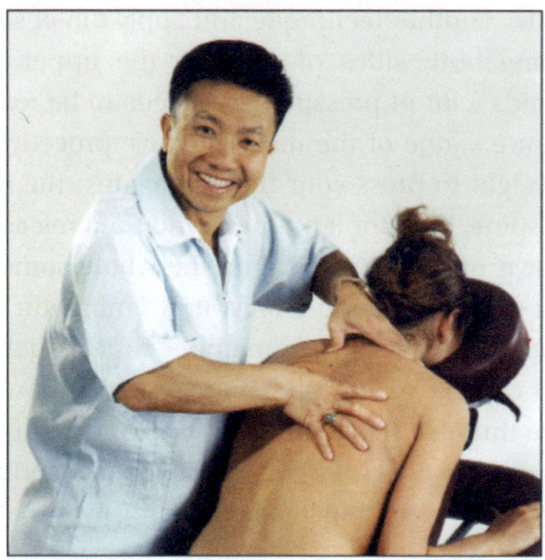

Kneading in a gentle rhythmic motion is a fantastic way to get energy flowing to the trapezius and levator scapulae muscles along the neck, shoulder blades and upper back. Rubbing this area will usually elicit appreciative noises from your partner.

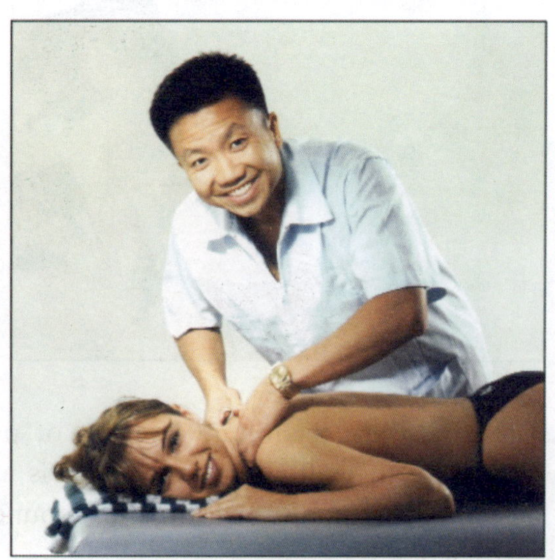

A gentle chopping with the side of the hands up and down the back muscles and across the trapezius and levator scapulae is another highly beneficial option. It is important not to "chop" too forcefully and to avoid the spinal column itself, because even a slight blow to the spine itself can cause harm. Concentrate this move on the muscles, not the bones.

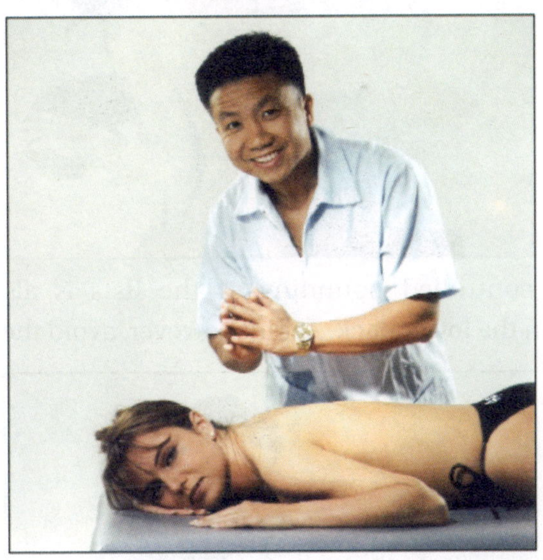

A variation of this is finger tapping, which offers a different frequency and vibration. Finger tapping is particularly pertinent to the upper back, where light stimulation is the best treatment. The technique involves just what it suggests: a gentle tapping of the muscles using the fingers, a bit like flattening dough for a pie or pizza crust. Another variation of this is to pat the back with the sides of your cupped hands.

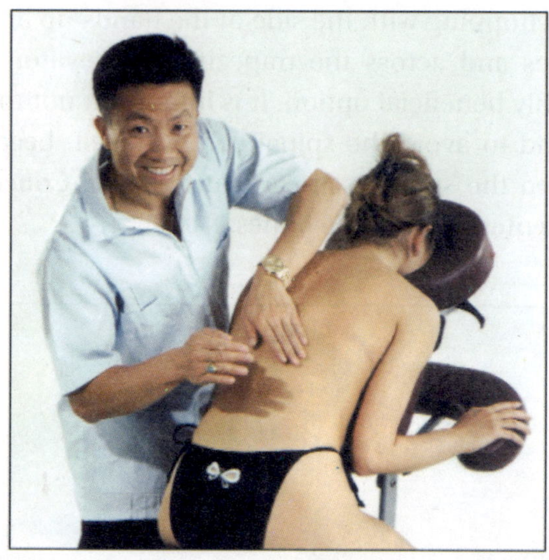

A light, controlled pounding of the fists is also effectual, especially on the lower back. Again, however, avoid the spine itself.

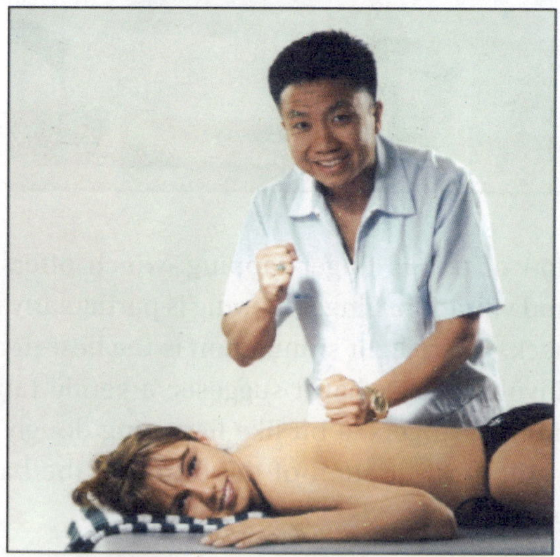

While studying acupuncture in China I picked up a move called the "knuckle roll" where you roll the knuckles over the surface of the back from side-to-side like a friction rub, which brilliantly warms the muscles and skin. This process is a little difficult to master, as the action comes from the elbow, but it is particularly great for the upper trapezius, where there is a lot of energy and pressure.

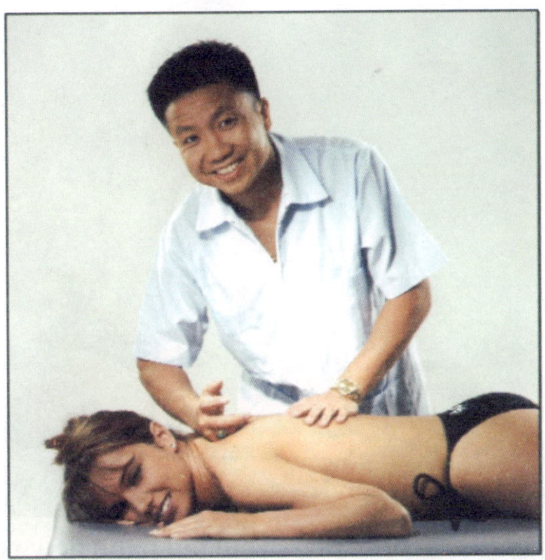

The masseuse can also gently "shake" the lower back by pushing it back and forth with the palms of the hands. This is a wonderful way to help your partner to passively loosen his or her spine.

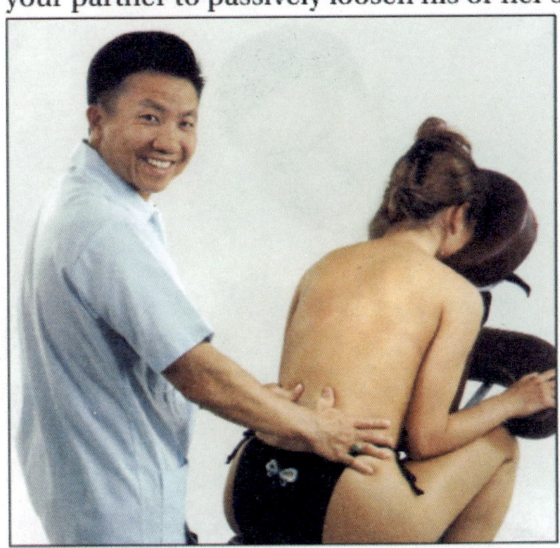

"Skin rolling" is a move wherein you lightly lift the skin running along the spine. You don't have to pull on it; just pick it up and let it drop. It's easy to do and it feels wonderful.

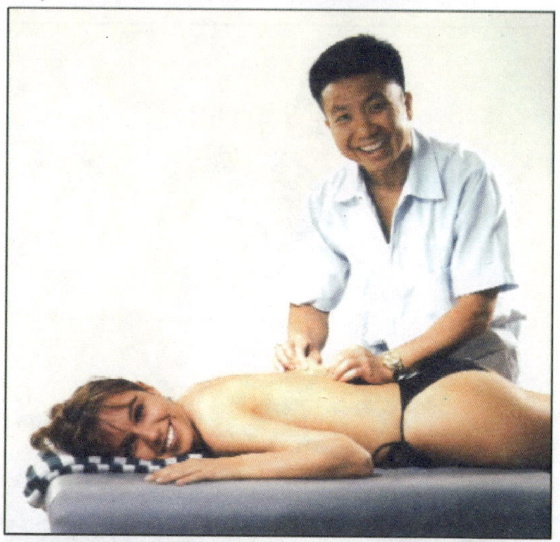

To apply gentle traction, press your left hand down on the lower back while pushing your right hand along the spine toward the head. This elongates the spine against the effects of gravity.

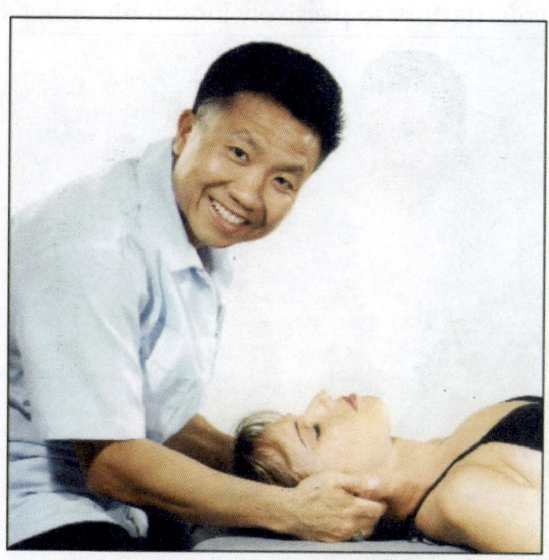

"Sculpting" refers to the dragging of hands along the back, which is an excellent way to finish off a massage. Perform this finale move for a few minutes, tapering the pressure until the person is completely relaxed.

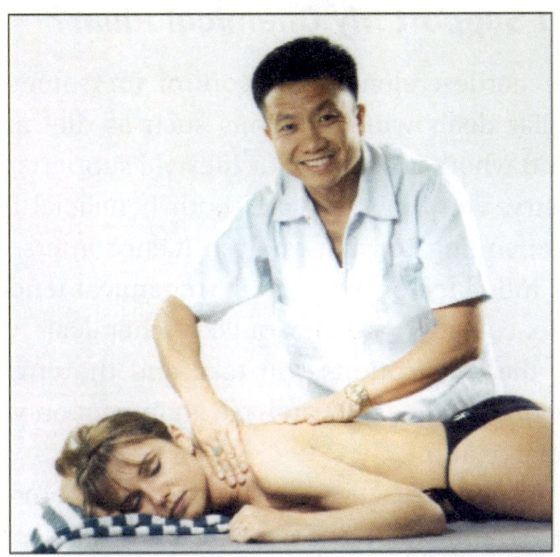

Once the massage is over, the subject should drink plenty of water to help flush out the toxins that were released from manipulated muscles.

Some words of caution: if you find an area on your subject that is tender or sore, I strongly advise that you stay away from it until the person has been to see a doctor. And it is very important to never massage a lump or other mass in a person's leg(s): doing so may release a clot that can be carried to the heart and cause dire consequences.

For those of you who may not have a willing partner, or who want more control over when and how often you can receive the benefits of massage, I strongly suggest that you try **TENS** therapy – a convenient, inexpensive and self-applied massage therapy you can do anytime and as often as you need, without having to lift a finger or learn a single massage technique. For more information, please see the section on **TENS**.

How Can I Support My Chemical Pillar?

Perhaps the hardest element to control for some people, the chemical pillar deals with functions such as diet and digestive processes and whether or not your lifestyle supports your brain's own chemistry. The brain releases both beneficial and harmful chemicals depending on what catalysts it encounters, and lifestyle has a direct influence on your brain's chemical tendencies. Also important to consider are the outside chemicals you may be exposed to, the medications you take and the environment in which you work and live. All can have an impact on your physical and emotional health.

Many people have reactions to some of the common chemicals in some foods and don't even realize it. Certain preservatives, artificial colours and flavours, additives and flavour enhancers like **MSG** can cause some people to experience headaches, nausea or have an irritable bowel. Quite simply, some foods don't agree with us and we ignore how they make us feel because we don't want to admit that our favourite Chinese dinner makes us feel slow or causes our heads to throb; or we pretend that the taco chips we ate at lunch had nothing to do with the stomach cramps we experienced a few hours later.

Almost any processed food (that includes most convenience foods, from fast food to boxed dinners to frozen entrees) contains chemical additives to enhance its flavour, extend its shelf life and/or to improve its colour or texture. You may be a perfectly healthy person and still suffer reactions to such chemicals and additives. And don't expect to be helped much by reading labels:

MSG (monosodium glutamate), which is a common additive used in Chinese food and most processed foods, causes reactions in some people, including migraine or tension headaches, dizziness and lethargy, but it is usually hidden within food labels under such vague terminology as "natural flavouring," "autolyzed yeast extract," "sodium caseinate," "maltodextrin," and others.

There are also a lot of unnamed chemicals in many meat products, including some of the innocent-looking poultry and steaks that you buy at the store. Many types of meat are cut and packaged using chemicals to enhance their flavour or to extend their shelf life. And of course, even good old fruits and vegetables are often sprayed with pesticides to discourage insects, and for some people these chemicals pose serious problems. Naturally it is important to always wash fruits and vegetables before you eat them, but even that may not be enough for someone who is sensitive to pesticide residue, especially on those items that have been "waxed" to make them look pretty, like apples and cucumbers.

So what's a person to do? If you ever have reactions to food (unexplained headaches, sleepiness, lethargy, gassiness or an irritable bowel), I strongly suggest that you begin keeping a food "diary." List everything you eat and where you got it (food store, restaurant, your own garden, etc.) and see if your food reactions involve a pattern that might pinpoint a food allergy, a chemical response or a possible intolerance to a certain variety of food, such as those containing lactose, like milk and ice cream. Begin excluding possible culprits one by one for at least two weeks and see if you find that you feel better. And if you think you're especially sensitive, I highly recommend that you cut out all processed foods entirely, in favour of a diet that involves more organic fruits and vegetables, fresh whole grains and other unprocessed, low-fat, high-fibre foods.

Other chemical reactions involve those that come from our

living environment: pollution, household products, poorly ventilated air and the general use of items that can produce an allergic reaction – from cleansers to cosmetics to shaving cream. Fragrances that make products more pleasant to use can also have adverse effects on sensitive people. If you find that inhaling your spouse's cologne or using a particular shampoo or household cleaner causes you to sneeze, have irritated eyes or gives you a dull headache, you are likely having a reaction to one of the many chemicals to which you're exposed every day. Some people can develop sensitivities to dyes, scents or compounds out of the blue, even though they've had no history of reaction to them before. And certain chemical mixtures, such as bleach and ammonia, are actually dangerous to breathe.

Outside pollution can be more difficult to control, but on days classified as poor-air days, try to stay inside as much as possible – especially if you are elderly or have any respiratory condition like asthma. Indoor pollution is another matter. You may suffer reactions from the insulation at your job or to the cleaning agent your dry cleaner uses to clean your clothes. If you have reason to believe that you suffer reactions to certain chemicals but aren't sure what they are, you can also keep of diary of the chemicals you are exposed to on a daily basis, as well as those physical environments that you find leave you feeling poorly – if you notice that you get a headache every time you enter the break room at work, for example, it may be reasonable to presume that a dirty air duct, the room's insulation or perhaps even a chemical they use to clean it or to prevent pests is causing you to have an adverse reaction. If there's nothing you can do to eliminate these chemicals from your life, the best thing to do is avoid them whenever possible.

Lastly, you will strengthen your body's struggles against the chemical and noxious pollution it encounters every day by drinking more water. Most people simply don't drink enough water – and they often compound the problem by drinking dehydrating liquids like coffee, tea or alcohol. The average person should drink at least 64 oz. (8 eight-oz glasses) every day, and even more if they weigh over 150 pounds. Water helps to flush toxins from our bodies better than anything else. By the way, there is no evidence that bottled water is any cleaner or more pure than municipally treated tap water – in fact, "luxury" water is less scrutinized and may contain more naturally occurring minerals that can make it taste strange to some people. Tap water can also contain strange flavours and have unwanted chemicals in it, such as chlorine and fluoride. Your best choice may be to invest in a good water filter or to buy distilled or purified water. They're typically cheaper per ounce than bottled waters and often taste better.

Another topic that I want to touch on but won't explore in detail due to the vastness of its scope is our own brain chemistry. Our brains secrete a variety of chemicals into our bodies on any given day: they control everything from whether we feel alert or sleepy, happy or sad, full of pain or pain-free. Many people in modern society take medication to help control imbalances in their brain chemistry and for some they are a miracle. It is my opinion, however, that some medications to treat certain maladies like depression are often over-prescribed for the same reason that painkillers are over-prescribed: it's easier and quicker for most MDS to give someone a pill and send them on their way than to go through the long and sometimes complicated ordeal of uncovering the roots of their problems. Again, this is too huge a topic to delve into within these pages, but please allow me to suggest that anyone who's been prescribed medication to treat an emotionally based problem should not look at such treatment as a cure-all. In your overall treatment you should always include methods that support you emotionally and address your *psycho-emotional pillar*.

How Can I Support My Psycho-Emotional Pillar?

This refers to your emotional or "spiritual" side. Are you often bombarded with negative feelings or emotional influences? How much stress do you face in the average day? Your attitude toward yourself and your health has a powerful influence on your ability to heal and feel good. Also of major importance is the support around you, whether it be from family, friends, co-workers, neighbours or the religious or spiritual community to which you may belong.

Probably most influential to your emotional health is your general feeling about yourself. Certainly we all have moments when we feel a bit foolish or unattractive or are affected by some other negative comment our inner voice makes when we're having a bad day or feeling insecure. These are normal (and irrational) thoughts that most people have from time to time and they usually pass. But for some of us, the feelings are present in the background of almost all the avenues of our lives – like distant echoes, they ricochet through our brains and leave us feeling exhausted, useless or hopeless. If you or someone you know fits this description, then it is likely that the problem is serious self-doubt issues. This is a very common problem, probably now more than ever because so many of us feel pressured to be perfect. "Failing" at being perfect (and every one of us is guilty of it, because not one of us is perfect), can make some people feel worthless. Such people tend to focus only on their inabilities and lose sight of their capabilities, their talents, their good nature, their generosity and all else that is wonderful about them.

If you find yourself having feelings of self-loathing, it is very important to seek emotional support. Don't delay, or the problem will only become more entrenched in your thinking. What the term "emotional support" means will be up to you, but start by choosing the most logical option and if it doesn't work after a reasonable try, move on to the next until you find a way to explore who you are and like what you find. Options include professional therapy, group therapy, talking openly with a kind and trusted friend or family member, religious outlets, guided meditation or even something like joining a club (such as a book or cooking club, or a club whose members may share a problem such as an illness) where you can meet others who share your interests and can offer you some support and acceptance.

Also important to your emotional well-being is to limit your exposure to the negative influences in your life. If you have a friend whom you find often leaves you feeling bad, maybe it's time to assess whether or not that person is still a friend. The same situation may apply to a family member, even your spouse – if there is anyone in your life whose influence feels more often bad than good, then consider taking steps to improve the environment. Of course, you will be the best person to decide what steps those should be, but don't ignore negativity in your life – do what you can to limit it as much as possible or change it for the better.

So what can we take away from reviewing the four pillars of health? The most important lesson is that by taking these individual components and viewing them as a whole, we can achieve optimal health. Contemplating all four pillars is what I refer to "looking at the whole body." It has served as the basis of my practice as a chiropractor and an acupuncturist, and I have learned to apply and continually improve upon it over my nineteen years of practice. By embracing different techniques and always keeping my mind open to new ones, I've managed to develop a complete and thorough approach to pain, one that incorporates the best elements of Western and Eastern cultures and the myriad approaches to healing – from traditional medicine to holistic therapies.

Merging Chiropractic and Acupunctural Teachings

I first became interested in helping people while working in my parents' family restaurant. In the service industry it is integral that you listen to your customers and respond to their needs. I've continued to maintain this view throughout my career as a chiropractor: healthcare begins and ends with the patient and his or her particular needs and wants. The role of the healthcare professional is to provide the best and most appropriate service and advice possible.

I feel fortunate to have been exposed to many different fields of health, technology and employment. Many healthcare professionals (and people in any profession) seem to have a tendency to dogmatically close their minds to everything except what they've learned in school. And often, the more specialized doctors become, the more closed and less helpful they become.

In my case, I've always liked to keep up on everything that interests me and might help me to help my patients. When I was about sixteen, friends of my grandmother's introduced me to acupuncture and I became fascinated with how even the most chronic pain conditions could be relieved through the insertion of fine needles – without drugs or surgery. I continued to pursue my interest and spent months training hands-on in Sri Lanka and China, and what I've learned through my years of study has become a central component of my chiropractic outlook.

Many MDS and chiropractors, unfortunately, are still unaware of the wonders of acupuncture because it hasn't been generally accepted as part of university curricula. Conversely, acupuncturists often think that their practice is the only path to healing. But I've found that chiropractic and acupunctural therapies are not contradictory – they in fact go hand-in-hand: the chiropractic approach addresses the mechanical aspect of the problem, such as whether it is situated in a joint or a muscle, while the acupunctural approach focuses on the flow of nerves and energy through the body.

The teachings of acupuncture are highly applicable to the chiropractic outlook. The general principle of acupuncture focuses on the energy that runs through your body in specific channels and the idea that if those channels are blocked or the flow is interrupted in any way, you can have pain that with time can develop into disease. The body has trouble healing itself until you remove the blockages and balance the flow. In chiropractic therapy, the basic principle is that your healing energy comes from your brain, goes down your spinal cord and branches out through the spine and spinal nerves. If your spine is not functioning properly, it can cause irritation of the nerves, which can then cause pain and create further dysfunction in the tissue that's being supplied by those nerves. The way to restore health is to restore the function of the spine by taking away any interference in the nervous system and allowing the body to heal itself.

So, you can see that the two have a lot of shared principles. From day one of my practice, I've advocated the marriage of the two schools of thought in treatment, and I've always received terrific results and feedback. It just makes common sense that different patients have different problems and many of them even have multiple problems from different sources. A close-minded cookie-cutter approach simply will not work if your goal is to offer effective treatment to as many people as possible.

The integration of these treatments, along with my interest in engineering, taught me that there are always ways of improving things. Ultimately my study of chiropractic therapy, acupuncture, medicine, physiotherapy, massage therapy and engineering, along with innumerable patient responses and feedback, led to my development of *Dr. Ho's Muscle Massage System*, a **TENS** therapy device that allows people to effectively treat their pain conditions in their own homes. And of the many accomplishments I've achieved in my pain practice, it may be the one of which I'm most proud.

What is TENS Therapy?

TENS stands for transcutaneous electrical nerve stimulation. What a good **TENS** device does is manipulate the muscles to cause deep tissue relaxation while promoting blood, lymphatic and nerve circulation. Just like traditional massage, **TENS** therapy can relieve pain, relax muscle spasm and promote faster healing.

There are many devices on the market that deliver electrical nerve stimulation to applied muscles – the ones you most likely have seen are those that claim to build "six-pack" abdominal muscles while you watch **TV** or relax in your recliner. There is no statistical or scientific evidence that **TENS** devices actually build muscle mass, so don't be tempted to waste your money on such promises. In fact, empirical evidence shows that such claims must be false, or else all my patients who have used **TENS** devices to treat sore muscles in their necks, backs and shoulders would look like linebackers or professional wrestlers.

What **TENS** therapy is ideally suited to do is to generate electrical stimulation patterns that cause distinct responses to applied muscle tissues: the nerves within these muscles receive increased circulation and react to the electrical impulses by causing the muscles to contract and expand again and again. Allowing these muscles to move and relax invites a number of beneficial things to happen:

- **Increased circulation** – *blood can fight its way past the barrier created by muscle tension and carry oxygen to the muscles and related soft tissues, relieving pain and allowing for tissue repair.*

- **Increased nerve conductivity** – *the nerves receive stimulation that allows them to properly service the muscles and relieves the nerves of chronic irritation and resulting limited or hyper-activity. Nerves that properly circulate function efficiently and cease creating hypersensitive responses. Proper circulation can also prevent damage to abnormally excited nerves that can cause numbness, weakness or slowed muscle response. Left untreated, such nerves can become permanently damaged.*

- **Allows for "gate control therapy"** – *gate control therapy is a simple way of describing what is called a presynaptic inhibition in the dorsal horn of the spinal cord. What this means is that electrical impulses delivered to the muscles may interrupt or confuse the pain signals' route from the spinal cord to your brain; if the signals don't reach the brain, your body won't recognize the signals and therefore won't release a pain response.*

- **Allows for flushing of noxious pain chemicals** – *when the brain gets pain or injury signals, it causes certain chemicals to be released in the affected (and sometimes distant) tissues that can become trapped by tight muscles, causing ongoing pain and furthering muscle tension. Relaxing the muscles through nerve stimulation helps to release these noxious chemicals so the tissue can be restored to full health and elasticity.*

- **Helps to stimulate the body's own endogenous pain controls** – *stimulation and relaxation of the muscles can promote the release of your body's own morphine-like painkillers* *called endorphins, enkephalins and dynorphins. These are the substances that make you feel good naturally and help you to resist pain mechanisms.*

- **Helps you to relax** – *TENS therapy can help relieve tension from all causes, including injury, immobility and emotional stress, all of which contribute to pain and other unwanted recurrent symptoms.*

Some of TENS therapy's other benefits are that it is exceptionally easy to use and quite inexpensive, especially over the long term. While traditional massage from a licensed therapist may indeed be relaxing and beneficial in some pain treatments, it is expensive therapy – the daily eight-week treatment that most people would require to train their muscles to relax would cost thousands of dollars, with subsequent treatments to offer preventive care costing many thousands more. And it falls short of TENS therapy in that it doesn't stimulate a muscle contraction/ relaxation response the way electrical stimulation will. The contraction/ relaxation response is key in helping to teach tense muscles to relax and to stop the spasm process. Further, traditional massage is also rather inconvenient, since it typically requires that one make appointments and travel to a clinic or salon. People who suffer frequent daily episodes involving pain, stiffness or numbness, or those who suffer at night, are seldom able to find appropriate massage treatment to allow for immediate relief using traditional massage therapies. In my years of studying TENS therapy, I've come to find that patients respond better over the long term to electrical nerve stimulation, also known as *electroanalgesia,* as a pain treatment than they do other forms of passive muscle therapy. TENS allows people to control when and how often they can receive treatment, so spasm and pain can be stopped as they happen, when treatment is most beneficial.

How Does a TENS Device Work?

A good TENS device should be small but powerful, and will deliver a variety of high and low frequency stimulation patterns for maximum benefit and relaxation capabilities. These patterns feel in many ways like a regular massage – they can range from soft and soothing to guided pulsing to a deep tissue massage. Which pulse pattern you pick depends entirely on what you need in a particular area on any given day. A good device will be completely portable and offer sufficient electrodes (the sticky, flexible pads that you place directly on your skin where pain exists) so that you can simultaneously stimulate the site of pain, for example your wrist, as well as the actual origination point of the pain – in this case, the C7 nerve at the junction of the neck and upper back. My study of various TENS devices quickly led me to the realization that they were all lacking: in power, in variability of pulse patterns, in effectiveness, in ease of use and/or in affordability. The final conclusion I came to was that if I wanted to be able to recommend such a device to my thousands of patients for their home use, that I had better develop my own: one that not only felt relaxing and pleasurable, but that would provide long-term and consistent pain relief. After thorough research and with the participation of and feedback from hundreds of patients suffering from a wide assortment of pain conditions, I perfected *Dr. Ho's Muscle Massage System* and made it available to not only the patients I see in my office, but to people all over the world who suffer from muscle tension-related maladies.

What Does It Feel Like?

Dr. Ho's Muscle Massage device provides gentle stimulation through varying electrical impulses. It feels like a deep, soothing hands-on massage, and is very relaxing. It features three different modes, each with at least four different simulated massage techniques, that are designed to relax tense muscles and to relieve pain. This variety of stimulation allows users to select the sensation they prefer and to adjust the intensity for maximum effectiveness and comfort. Most people will experience a sense of deep relaxation, reduction in their muscle tension and pain, and improvement in their blood and nerve circulation within only twenty minutes of treatment. With this portable home-care device, the longer and more frequently you use it, the better and faster your rate of recovery from many common painful conditions.

The modes perform as follows:

Mode one *simulates a massage sensation similar to thumb and palm kneading, finger tapping, soothing squeezing and variable-speed deep vibration. These medium-intensity techniques feel like a real hands-on massage. This mode is highly preferred by most users.*

Mode two *simulates a deeper, penetrating type of technique. It's more like a light flat-handed chopping motion followed by a mild pounding before proceeding to a variable-speed oscillation and, finally, a shaking type of sensation. Mode two is for the user who likes a very strong, deep massage.*

Mode three *is for someone who is more sensitive. This user typically prefers a lighter, more superficial rub. Mode three also comes in handy when you want to apply the device to an area where you probably want a very gentle stimulation, such as the face. Mode three graduates from a gentle rubbing on the skin with a little tingling underneath, to the sensation of someone gently but continuously gripping your muscles, to the lifting of the muscles with hands before letting the muscles completely relax.*

Within each mode, the stimulation will alternate randomly to prevent you and your nervous system from adapting. This unique feature of *Dr. Ho's Muscle Massage System* assures that you will get immediate and long-term relief for your painful condition(s).

We deliberately grouped the machine's stimulation variations so that you can easily select the sensation and type of massage you feel most comfortable with. This feature enables you to have an enjoyable massage and a more relaxing experience. Everybody has a favourite mode. The result is the same no matter which mode you use, and experienced users often end up mixing the three modes because they develop an appreciation for cycling through the different sensations.

Does TENS Therapy Really Work?

There are literally hundreds of clinical reports about the use of TENS therapy for different pain conditions, as well as other types of conditions such as bladder incontinence. Many of these reports are somewhat flawed because they are based on uncontrolled studies and because there are no uniform guidelines about what features a TENS device must have to be considered appropriate for use on these conditions. Quite frankly, some TENS devices I've encountered are flimsy, deliver weak pulse signals that offer limited stimulation to muscles and nerves, produce unpleasant sensations, or are difficult to use. Many offer only one treatment surface, or treatment pads of illogical sizes, so that balanced stimulation to an area – an important component of TENS treatment – is impossible.

The results of independent laboratory studies involving adequate TENS devices, however, suggest that there is solid clinical evidence that **TENS** therapy actually reduces pain by limiting the pain transmissions that reach the brain. Transmissions that get rerouted on their way from the spinal cord to the brain end up somewhat like a very weak radio signal – they may still exist, but their signals are so weak that they go totally ignored. And when the body is able to ignore these signals, it doesn't release the noxious chemicals, nor the signals to muscles to protect themselves by constricting, nor other undesirable responses that lead to pain and an increased vulnerability to injury. So not only can proper **TENS** therapy help relieve pain and assist in the healing of soft tissues, but it may also help prevent injury and reinjury to prone tight muscles, ligaments and tendons. Clinical studies specifically support **TENS** therapy as an effective treatment for many conditions, such as joint pain from rheumatoid arthritis and osteoarthritis, post-traumatic pain, menstrual pain, facial pain, brachial plexus avulsion, pain after spinal cord injury, angina pectoris and urge incontinence, as well as for patients requiring dental anaesthesia. These reports also discuss the positive results of using of **TENS** to assist patients in regaining motor function following strokes.

Of course, I wanted an independent source to study *Dr. Ho's Muscle Massage System*, to compare it with others on the market and also to verify what I already knew. The study, conducted by Stuart M. McGill, Ph.D., who is the Professor of Spine Biomechanics at the University of Waterloo, Ontario, produced the following findings:

> *"Our work shows that the sophisticated modulated patterns of Dr. Ho's stimulation device reduces muscle spasm and increases oxygenation, suggesting that the pain-spasm cycle is reduced." Conclusion: "A treatment consisting of muscle stimulation with [this] novel device while relaxing in a lying posture reduces pain, which*

may be due to the observed reduction in spasm and increase in muscle oxygenation."[2]

Dr. Ho's Muscle Massage System is clinically and scientifically proven to:

1. *Dramatically reduce muscle tension and muscle spasms.*
2. *Increase the oxygen level in the tissues during and after treatment.*
3. *Dramatically relieve pain and stiffness.*
4. *Increase muscle strength and tone.*
5. *Increase the range of movement in the neck, shoulder and lower back.*

Through self-adhesive electrodes attached to the skin, *Dr. Ho's Muscle Massage* device generates a gentle electrical pulse that stimulates the nerves and muscles by reproducing the twelve different types of soothing and relaxing massage techniques. It automatically varies the type of stimulation every few seconds in order to prevent your body from adapting and becoming immune to a particular modality. As a result, your muscles and nerves learn to relax and restore their healthy tone much faster. By forcing the appropriate receptors to induce relaxation, the machine essentially retrains muscles to stay relaxed. Calm muscles reduce irritation of the nerves and blood vessels, thereby encouraging blood and nerve circulation to increase the amount of oxygen at the tissue level, boost natural healing and enhance the removal of waste metabolites. Who knew that something that feels so good is also so beneficial?

[2]*Description and Comparison of Traditional T.E.N.S. to Dr.-Ho's T.E.N.S.*, Stuart M. McGill, PhD; June 2002.

Situations Where TENS Therapy is Not Advised

- *TENS therapy is **not** appropriate for use over the anterior (front) of the neck because it can cause spasm of the laryngeal muscles.*

- *TENS should **not** be used by anyone with a pacemaker.*

- *TENS should **not** be used during any stage of pregnancy because it can induce premature labour.*

- *TENS should **not** be applied over the carotid sinuses.*

- *The electrodes should **not** be placed in an area of sensory impairment (nerve lesions, neuropathies, etc.) or on skin that has been burned.*

- *A TENS unit should be used cautiously by patients who have a spinal cord stimulator or intrathecal pump. If you use such devices, first consult with your doctor about the appropriateness of TENS therapy.*

Treating Specific Injuries and Pain Conditions

In addition to the general daily stretching and exercise treatments that I recommend for reducing, limiting and preventing pain disorders associated with neck and upper back muscle tension, these treatments are designed to help pinpoint specific pain conditions and address them successfully. For each condition, I will provide my opinion as to the most plausible cause, the recommended treatment method using *Dr. Ho's Muscle Massage System*, and specially designed exercises that will assist you in getting immediate and long-term relief. It is my wish that when your body starts to function better and when you can live without your daily aches and pain, you will enjoy life to the fullest. Some general rules for using a **TENS** device include:

1. *For any painful condition, each treatment should be at least twenty minutes each time. You can treat yourself three to six times per day or as needed. Don't worry about overusing it — it is safe to use as often as you need it.*

2. *Always position your body in a neutral and relaxed posture for best results.*

3. *If you suffer from any upper extremity condition, I recommend that you also treat your neck because you may have a dysfunction there that could prevent your upper extremity problem from getting better.*

General Treatment for Neck Pain and Stiffness

General neck pain is most likely caused by excessive muscle tension in the neck. The contracted muscles will also cause restriction in joint movement, restriction in blood flow and irritation of nerves that exit from the neck. Whatever the cause of the pain and tension, the appropriate home treatment will help speed your recovery. Temporary use of non-steroidal anti-inflammatory drugs (**NSAIDs**) such as Aspirin, Advil or Aleve may help relieve pain from injury or strain, but should be used for no longer than a few days. If you can, it is often best to avoid them altogether in favour of the following therapies:

- **Ice.** *Place an ice pack or cold pack (in a pinch a package of frozen vegetables will work) over painful muscles for ten to fifteen* *minutes at a time, as often as once an hour. This will help decrease any pain, muscle spasm or swelling. If the problem is near the shoulder or upper back, ice the back of the neck.*

- **Movement.** *Return to your normal daily activities as soon as possible. Continuing normal activities helps relieve more symptoms than taking leave from work and using neck immobilization therapies such as cervical collars.*

- **Avoidance.** *Avoid activities that may be causing your neck pain, such as prolonged computer work or overhead work like painting or woodworking — or at least change or restructure how you do them.*

- **Stretch, exercise and maintain good posture.** *Move your neck side to side gently every half an hour to maintain fluid movement and to restore range of motion. Follow my complete movement and exercise routine laid out earlier in this chapter.*

- **Implement Regular Massage.** *Have someone gently massage your neck, scalp, shoulders and/or back to relax tight muscles. Or better yet, use a TENS device such as Dr. Ho's Muscle Massage System to restore normal function in your neck. If you have a history of injuries or if your job causes excessive strain on your neck muscles, use the device daily to prevent tension buildup.*

Using Dr. Ho's Muscle Massage Device on Tense Neck Muscles

1. *Lie on your back with a rolled-up heavy towel, sponge roll or a firm orthopedic pillow under your neck.*

2. Place pads over the most tense area(s) of the neck.

3. Perform deep abdominal breathing.

Note: *Do not stimulate the front of the neck.*

To restore maximum range of motion in your neck, use *Dr. Ho's Muscle Massage System* and perform the neck rotation exercise on a daily basis. Gently rotate your neck side to side ten times each side within your comfort range every thirty minutes daily till you reach maximum recovery.

Can I Use TENS to Treat Sports Injuries?

While some serious sports injuries need surgical intervention, most will respond well to treatments that can relax the muscles quickly and stimulate nerve and blood circulation. Massage therapy, chiropractic therapy and physiotherapy all work to relax the muscles and restore alignment and movement in the joints. Most sports therapy clinics utilize electrical modalities to relieve pain while stimulating faster tissue repair. In fact, one of the most effective methods for stimulating nerve and blood circulation while reducing muscle tension and relieving pain is through the application of electrotherapy stimulation. Many chiropractors, massage therapists, physiotherapists and other sports injury specialists use TENS to help reduce muscle tension, relieve pain and stimulate blood and nerve circulation.

Dr. Ho's Muscle Massage System represents a new class of electrotherapy machines. Because the device is programmed to randomly change its output in order to prevent adaptation by the nervous system, it is a vast improvement on the larger, more expensive traditional TENS machines that all send out a steady impulse. *Dr. Ho's Muscle Massage* device is extremely effective in maintaining muscle tone and for treating a variety of sports-related injuries. Many amateur and professional athletes use it: after other forms of therapy failed them, Major League Baseball all-star Gary Sheffield and National Hockey League player Brad May have both experienced incredible recoveries from its use. *Dr. Ho's Muscle Massage System* is proven to provide immediate and long-term relief for many types of sports-related injuries including neck and shoulder pain, lower back pain and many other muscle-strain and ligament-sprain related syndromes.

Treating Pain from RSDs, Injury and Disease

Whatever the cause of your pain, treating it using massage and TENS therapy is materially the same for all, so you will find them catalogued here not by cause but by where the pain is felt, making it easy to navigate your path to relief.

Most acute and chronic muscle pain and RSD-related injuries will respond well to treatments that can relax the muscles quickly and stimulate nerve circulation. Massage therapy, chiropractic therapy and physiotherapy all work to relax the muscles and restore alignment and movement in the joints of the neck and upper back.

People who sit or lift excessively should implement daily massage of their lower backs, hips and the backs of their legs to treat and prevent lower back pain, hip pain and poor leg circulation due to pinched sciatic nerve(s) or stagnation of blood flow.

Proper treatment also includes therapy to minimize inflammation and development of scar tissue while maintaining blood flow to the overused tendon(s). To facilitate greater nerve conduction, blood circulation and muscle response, you can easily treat your condition(s) at home using a **TENS** device such as *Dr. Ho's Muscle Massage System.* All you need to do is identify where the pain is and treat it at the site of pain, as well as the neck area where the pain most likely begins. Here is a list of the pain sites and the probable sources, where indicated, that usually originate in the neck. Use them as a reference for your **TENS** treatment, and also note the applicable exercises to strengthen the affected area(s).

Upper Shoulder Pain

Upper shoulder pain is most likely caused by muscle tension in the shoulders and in the neck at the C7-C8 nerves. This can lead to shoulder tension, neck pain and headaches.

You can treat the upper shoulder muscles while sitting upright or lying on your back.

Place one pad on each side of the upper shoulders and the upper trapezius muscles.

Many people have a painful spot just beside the shoulder blade. You can position one electrode on this painful spot and have the second electrode on the upper shoulders, or use all four pads to create symmetry on all spots. I suggest that you use *Dr. Ho's Muscle Massage System* after spending long hours on the computer or while doing other stationary activities.

The best way to strengthen the upper shoulders is by doing push-ups. If you haven't done push-ups in awhile, you should start by doing them standing up against a counter with your body angled. Start by doing ten in the morning and ten again before bedtime.

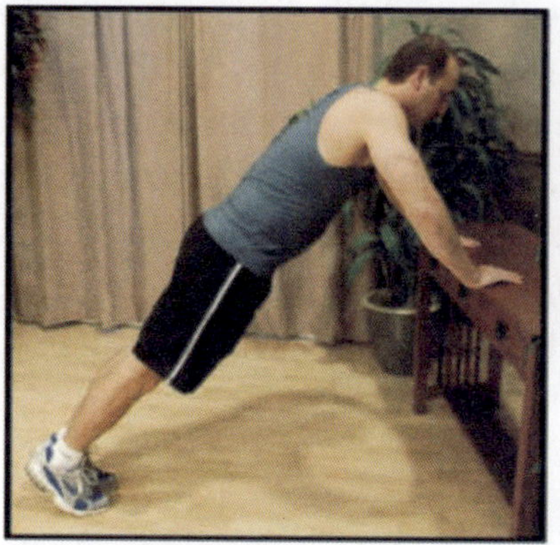

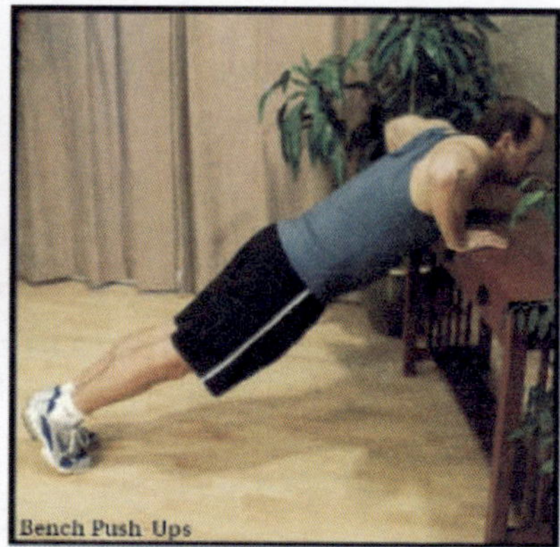

Bench Push-Ups

When you are able to do thirty push-ups without straining, then increase the resistance by doing the push-ups on the floor. Depending on your strength, you can perform push-ups on your knees or toes. Pace yourself as your upper shoulders become stronger with regular exercise.

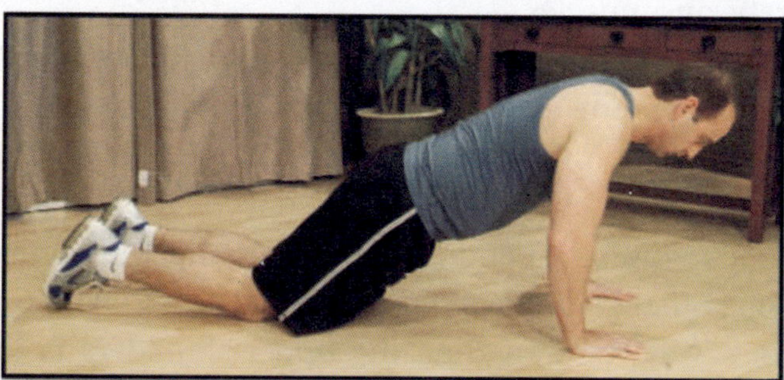

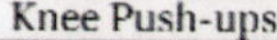

Knee Push-ups

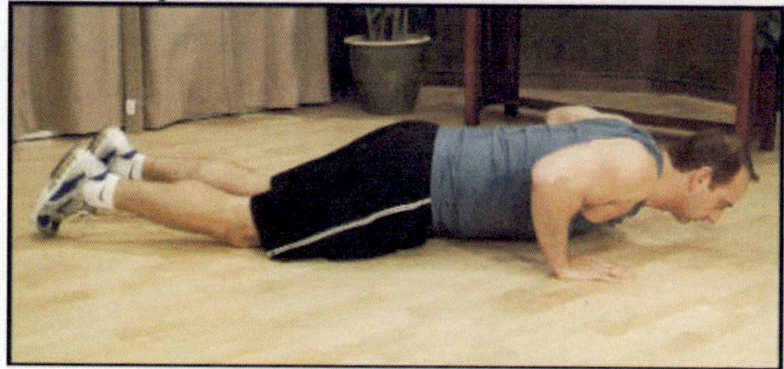

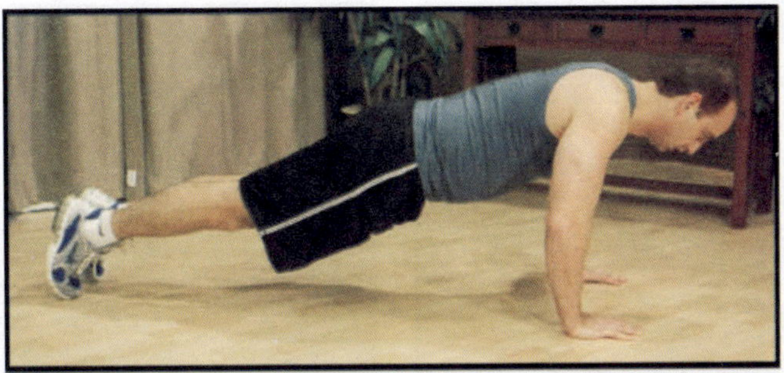

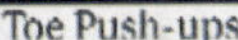
Toe Push-ups

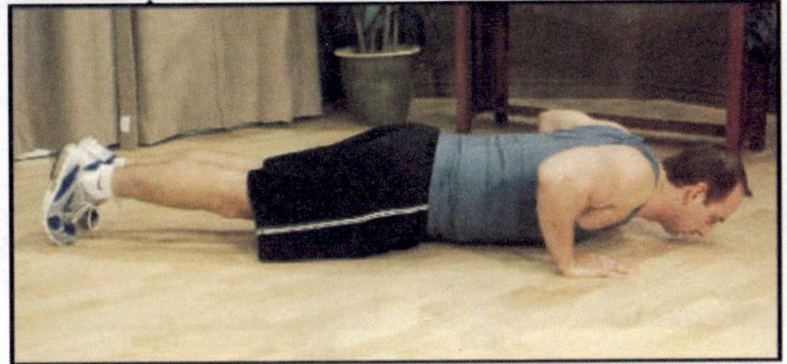

Shoulder Joint Pain

The shoulder joint is one of the weakest joints in the human body. Shoulder pain is usually related to bursitis, arthritis and rotator cuff tendinitis.

Sit comfortably in a chair with your affected arm resting on a cushion or pillow on your lap. Place one electrode in front of and another behind the shoulder joint. Treat this area for ten to twenty minutes and then place the electrodes on the top and side of the shoulder for another ten to twenty minutes of treatment. Or use all four pads at once to treat the areas simultaneously.

Perform shoulder windmill exercises. Start with the arm up, rotate downward rapidly and let the momentum carry the shoulder around, followed by the other arm. Perform these ten times forward and then backward three to four times a day.

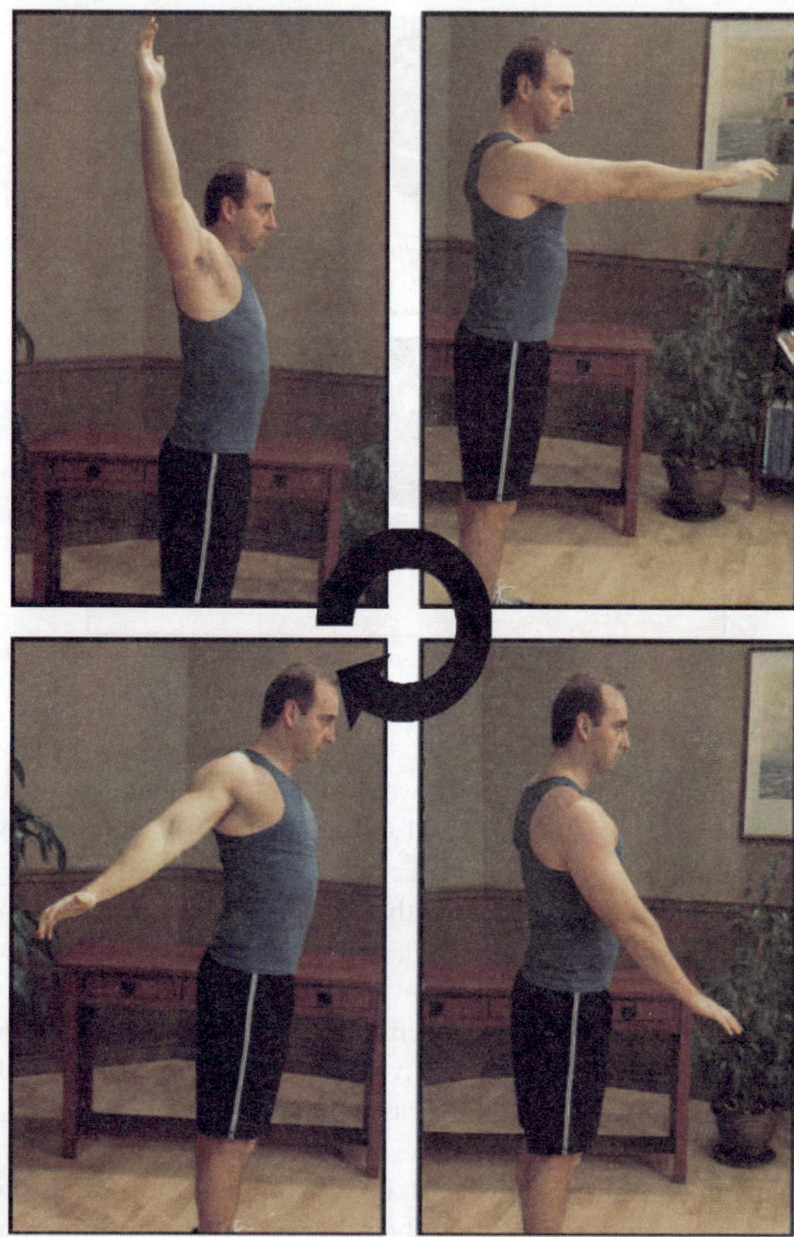

Note: shoulder pain that fails to get better with the above treatment may indicate that the nerves from the neck are irritated. In order for your shoulder to heal, you have to relax the neck muscles and take the pressure off the nerves that run from your neck to your shoulder. I recommend that you treat your neck with any upper extremity condition because you can have a dysfunction in your neck that could prevent your problem from getting better. In most cases of shoulder pain, the culprits are the C5 and C6 nerves situated at the lower neck.

Elbow Pain

Elbow pain is usually related to lateral epicondylitis (tennis elbow) or medial epicondylitis (golfer's elbow). In both cases, the source of pain at the neck is most often the C7 and/or C8 nerves, as well as the T1.

Sit comfortably in a chair with the affected arm resting on a table or on a pillow on your lap. Place one electrode on the painful spot and the second electrode just below that spot on back of the arm for tennis elbow. Do the same treatment on the palm side for golfer's elbow. Treat the area(s) for ten to twenty minutes as often as needed.

Forearm exercise: In order to take pressure off the elbow, it is important to relax and lengthen the forearm muscles. To gently stretch the forearm muscles, you can do the following exercise: with your palm facing you, grip the hand with your opposite hand and then straighten your elbow while keeping the palm facing your chest. Repeat this ten times.

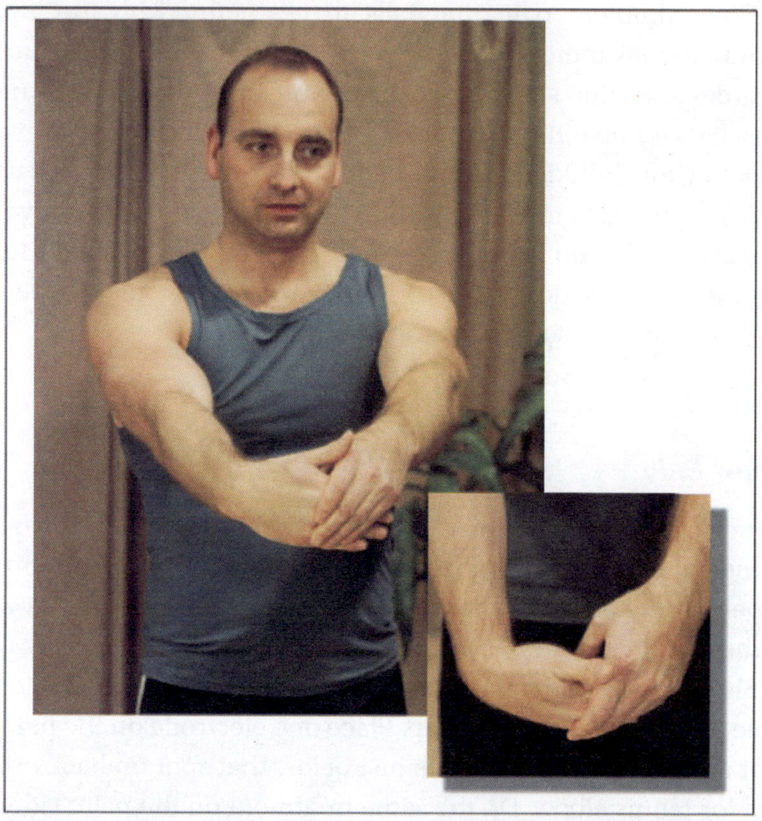

Now flip your palm to face away from your chest and straighten your elbow while keeping your palm away from your chest. Your opposite hand will provide resistance. Repeat ten times. Perform these forearm stretching exercises ten times every three to four hours throughout the day.

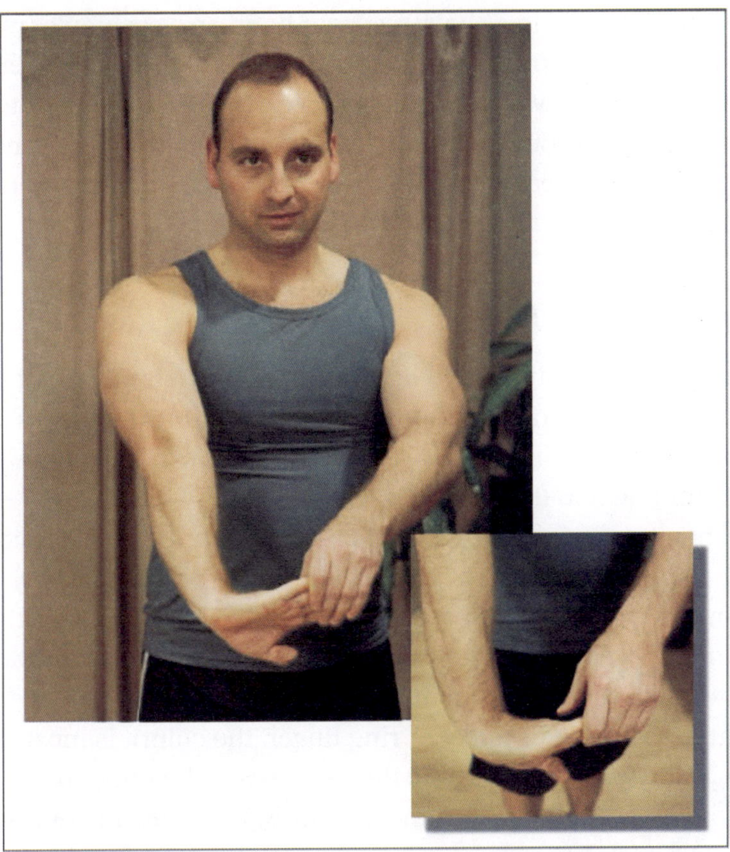

Wrist Pain

Wrist pain and tension can be instigated by excessive use and poor ergonomics. More commonly, wrist pain, numbness, pain and weakness in the wrist and the hand are related to the C7 and/or C8 nerves being irritated in the neck. These irritated nerves become swollen and painful as they go through the carpal tunnel in the wrist.

Use *Dr. Ho's Muscle Massage System* on the wrist, forearm and the lower neck/upper back for the most effective treatment plan.

Sit comfortably in a chair; rest your hand on a cushion or pillow on your lap. Place one electrode on each side of the wrist. With this treatment, you may feel an energy surge going from the wrist to the hand. This will promote conduction and circulation of the nerves. You should also treat your lower neck and do the forearm exercises detailed in the previous section on elbow pain.

Hand and Finger Pain

Hand pain is usually due to osteoarthritis or rheumatoid arthritis of the joints. Referral pain from irritated C7 and/or C8 nerves from your neck or the T1 nerve in your upper back can also cause pain and numbness in the hands.

When treating your fingers, place one electrode on each side of your finger to "sandwich" the painful joint. Sit comfortably in a chair, rest your hand on a cushion or pillow on your lap. If you suffer tenosynovitis of the thumb or forefinger, it is also important to treat the C7 nerve at the base of the neck. If the pain or numbness is in your pinky or ring finger, the culprit is most likely the C8 and/or T1 nerve where the neck meets the upper back.

To increase the range of movement in the joints in your hand, mobilize each finger by gently and repeatedly moving the fingers their complete range of movement. The more you do this passive mobilization exercise, the more movement you will restore in the stiff joints.

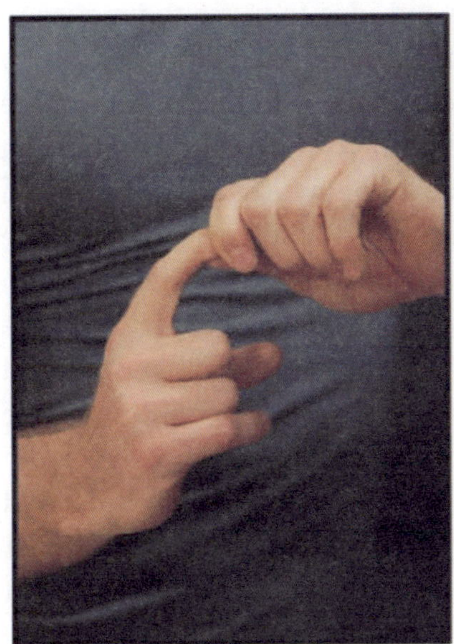

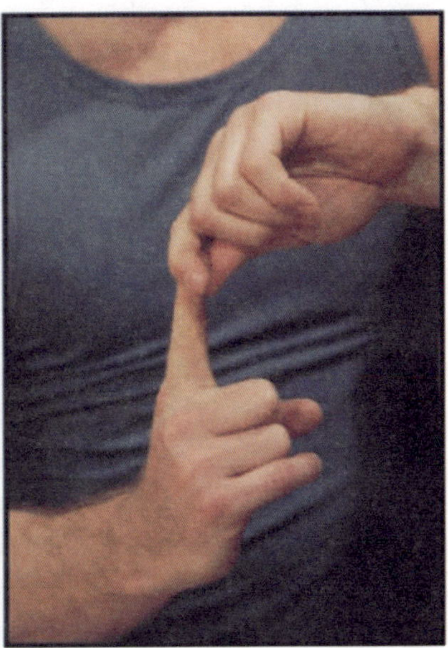

Tips to Help Avoid RSDs

Proper body mechanics can help most people avoid repetitive stress disorders, including taking frequent breaks and avoiding repetitive movements that involve a twisted or bent wrist (typing, use of certain tools and driving are typical causes). Stretching of the hands during periods of hand/ wrist activity is very important, as is varying the way you do anything you must do often, and trying to avoid tensing the hands or wrists whenever possible.

Our computer age has ushered in more complaints of wrist, forearm and hand pain, as more people are now required to type at least some in order to use desktop, laptop and hand-held devices. It is common for people to notice pain only on their "dominant" side, since that is often the hand and wrist that manipulates the mouse. Even as little as half an hour of constant "mousework" over the course of a few days or weeks can create injury in some.

Therefore, when possible, it is a good idea to move the mouse to different locations so your hand and wrist get a variety of movement. Cordless mouse devices make variety easier than the traditional kind because they're easier to move and respond on almost any surface – you can place them in different positions on your desk. People may also be in inhospitable environments like poorly designed workstations or workstations they share with others who are not the same weight or height. People are more prone to injury when they repeat movements with elbows held off to the side or when they rest elbows on armrests or on desks while working. Wrists, too, need proper placement and should remain straight, not arched. While typing in particular, hands should "float" over the keyboard – the wrists should never rest on it. For every few minutes of typing, you should extend your arms in front of you and wiggle your fingers. Now shake your arms loosely, allowing your fingers to flop around and your hands to go completely loose as you shake them. Actually, it's sort of fun – you may feel a little silly doing it, but you don't have to leave your desk and it will instantly increase circulation to stressed areas.

Other Common Pain Sites

Mid-back Pain

Mid-back pain is related to muscle tension in your neck and to the movement of your rib cage. Most people will note a pain spot just beside the shoulder blade. This problem can be aggravated by the slumped posture many people take during work.

You can treat this by placing one electrode directly over the painful spot and the second electrode on the lower neck area. Ideally, you should be lying down with your neck supported by a rolled-up towel or an orthopedic pillow. You can also treat yourself while sitting up in a high-back chair.

To restore movement in your rib cage, you'll need to perform a rib cage motion exercise. Bring both your elbows back while taking a very deep breath to expand your rib cage. Then push your arms forward while exhaling to deflate your rib cage. This is what I call an "air push-up." Repeat this ten times every thirty minutes daily until your mid-back pain is gone. You should also be doing the push-up and neck rotation exercises I described earlier.

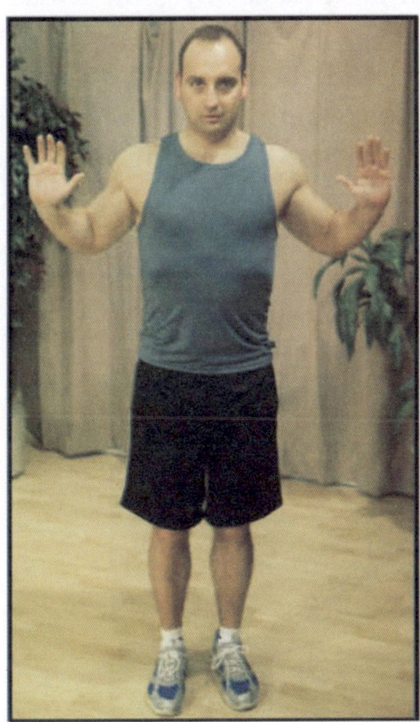

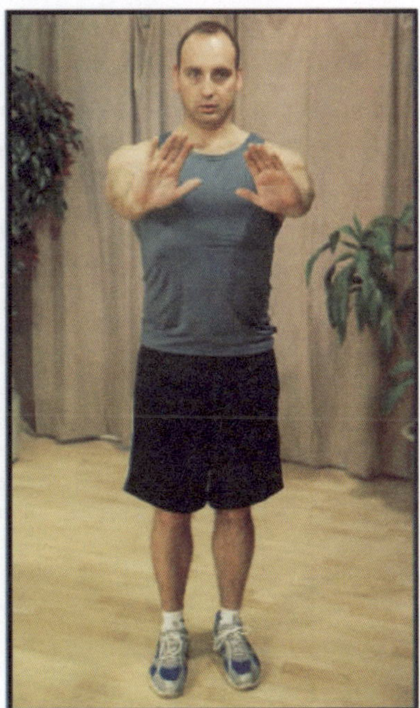

Lower Back Pain

Lower back pain can be caused by muscle tension, joint stiffness, herniated discs and/or irritated nerves – singularly or in combination.

To treat your lower back pain, sit in a comfortable chair with good back support. Sit way back until your buttocks and lower back touch the back of the chair. Place one electrode on the painful spot on your lower back and the second electrode on your hip, or use all four pads to treat both legs and hips simultaneously. I recommend that you treat both the lower back *and* the hip even if pain exists in only the lower back. It is important to treat the hip area because this is where the sciatic nerve exits and travels down the leg. *Be sure that you're sitting back and that the pads are pressed tightly against your skin.*

Back exercise: Keep your back muscles loose by gently twisting your lower back from side to side. To do this properly, start the twist by swinging your arms to one side, then turn your head and the rest of your spine will follow. Make sure that you're standing with your feet comfortably apart. Focus on relaxing your back muscles during the twist. Twist from one side to the other side ten times every thirty minutes to one hour throughout the day.

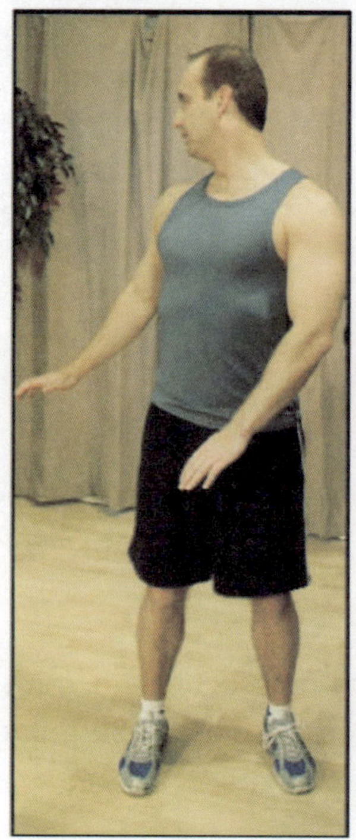

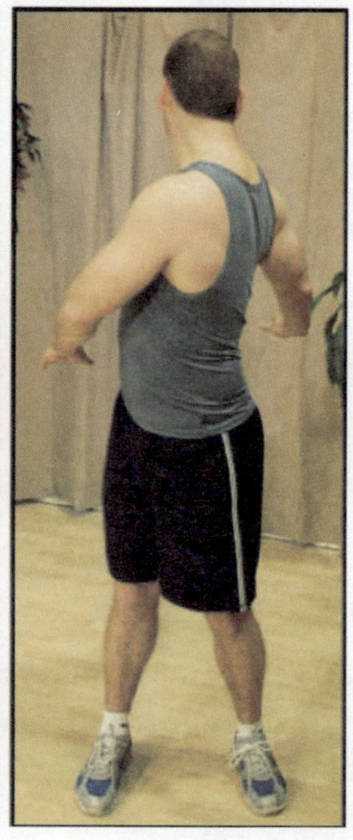

Another exercise that will help is to lie on your back and then pull one knee up toward the opposite shoulder, hold for ten seconds and then do the same on the other side. Perform the knee to opposite shoulder stretch each morning and before going to bed.

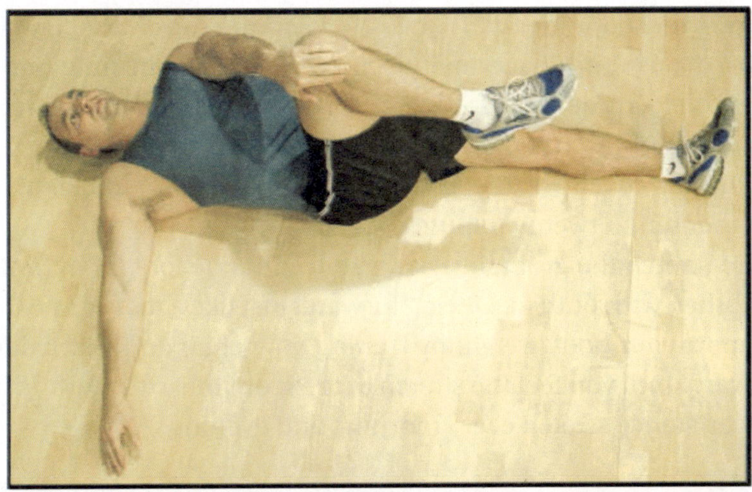

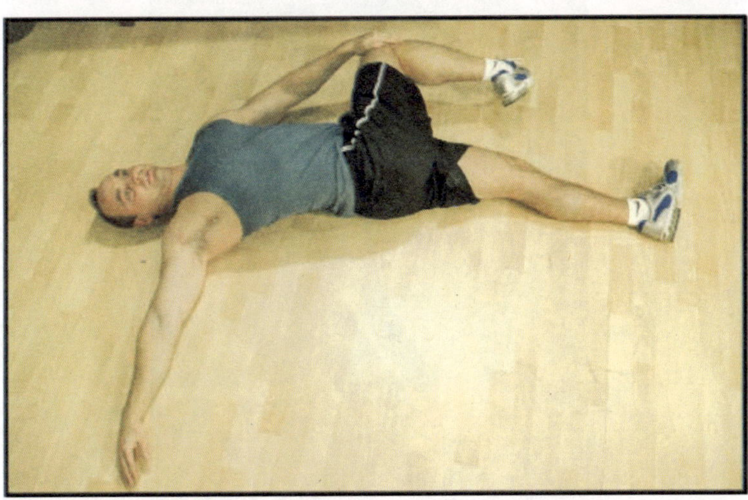

Groin Pull

Groin muscles can be strained by flexing the hip vigorously during sports activities. Overstretching of the muscles in the groin causes painful groin pulls that can make moving around unbearable.

To treat the groin muscles, lie on your back with two large pillows tucked under your knees to keep the hips flexed and in a relaxed position. Place one electrode at the groin line and the second electrode below the groin line. Treat this area for ten to twenty minutes and then move the electrode that was below the groin line to above the groin line. Repeat the stimulation for another ten to twenty minutes.

To stretch the groin muscles, stand with one foot far in front of the other, with both feet facing forward, just like a fencer's posture. Support your body weight by leaning on a chair and slowly lunge forward until you feel the stretch at the groin muscles. Perform the fencer-stance stretch every morning and evening.

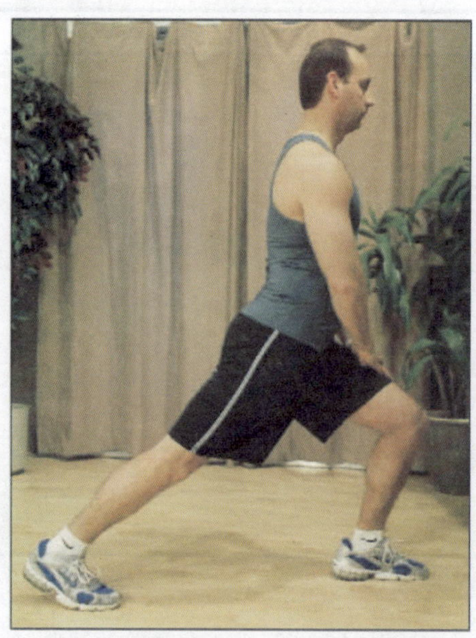

Hip Pain

Pain in the hip or buttock can be caused by osteoarthritis of the hip joint, referral pain from the lower back, or tension in the lower back and hip.

You can treat the hip by either sitting upright in a chair with back support or lying on your abdomen with a pillow beneath your pelvis.

Place one electrode at your mid-buttock and another on the painful spot on your hip. If you think that the hip pain might be related to your lower back, then you should treat the lower back as described above.

To loosen up the hip joint and stretch the muscles of the hip, gently swing the hip from front to back like a pendulum. You should also perform the knee-to-shoulder stretch exercise I prescribe for the lower back.

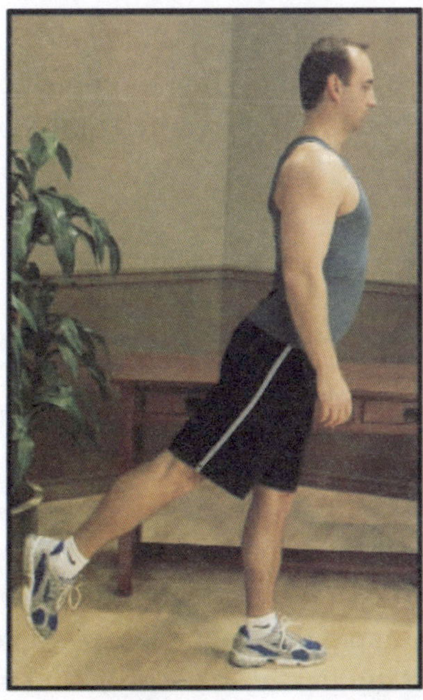

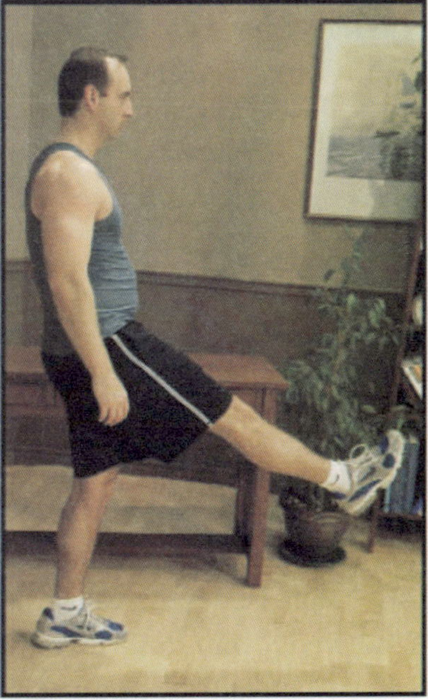

Sciatica

Sciatica is a pain that runs along the pathway of the sciatic nerve, from your lower back through your hip and then down your leg. The leg pain is the result of the nerve being irritated by tight muscles in your lower back and hip. A bulging lumbar disc can also cause sciatica by putting pressure on the nerve.

Initially, you can use the same treatment I recommend for lower back and hip pain. Place one electrode on the lower back and the second on the hip area. Treat yourself for at least ten to twenty minutes at a time, three to six times per day. This treatment will take pressure off the nerve and the lumbar discs. If the pain or numbness is not gone after about half an hour, leave one electrode on the buttock area and place the second electrode on the back of the knee. If your sciatica goes down to your toes, place the second pad on the bottom of your foot while leaving the other electrode on your hip.

Do the same exercise I suggest for the lower back and hip in the morning and before bedtime. Perform the knee-to-opposite-shoulder stretch, hold for a count of ten, and repeat ten times on each side.

Knee Pain

Knee pain is commonly caused by osteoarthritis, rheumatoid arthritis and sports injuries.

When treating your knee pain, sit comfortably in a chair with both your feet placed flat on the ground. Alternatively, you can lie on your back and support the back of your knee with two large pillows to keep it bent. Place one electrode on each side of the knee on the depressed area just beside the kneecap. Treat this area for ten to twenty minutes. After that, apply the electrodes to where you have pain and treat yourself for another ten to twenty minutes.

Passive knee movement: Throughout the day, gently swing your knee back and forth in a pendulum-like motion. If you have cartilage that is partially worn out, you should build up to a point where you're swinging your knee(s) about two thousand times per day – yes, the more the better. This passive swinging motion will lubricate the knee joint and bring in nourishment for the cartilage to promote regeneration.

When you combine the passive treatment with the TENS treatment of *Dr. Ho's Muscle Massage* device, the cartilage of your knee will become smooth and less painful over time.

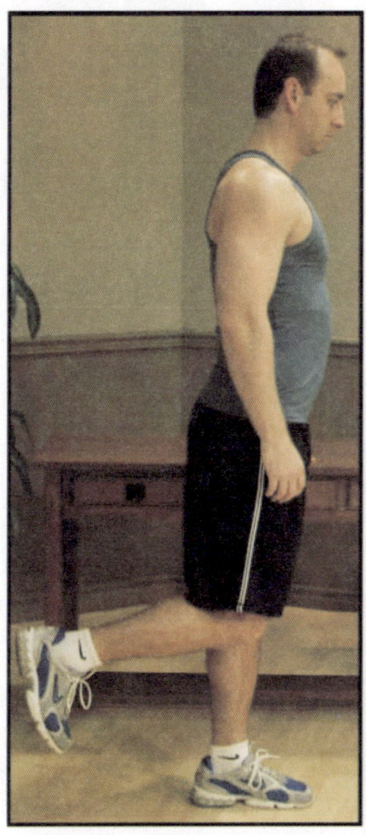

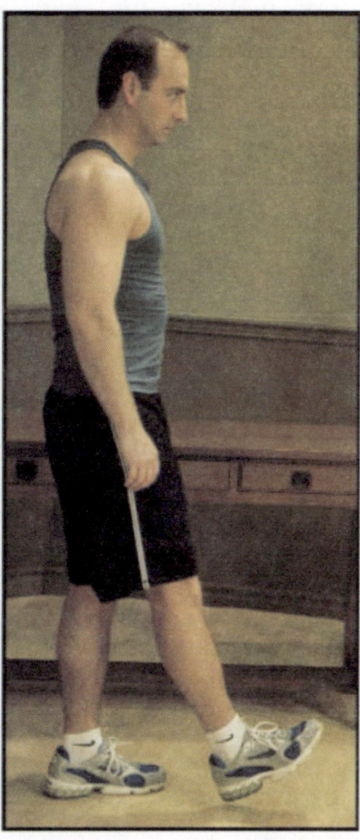

Thigh Muscle Strain

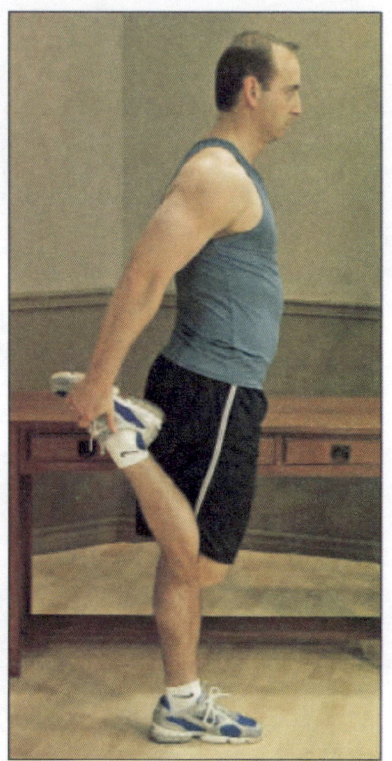

Thigh muscles are usually strained from overexertion during sports or other physical activities that you don't perform on a routine basis.

To treat your thigh muscles, lie on your back with two pillows under your knees to keep the knees flexed and the thigh muscles in a loose and relaxed position. Place one pad over the centre of the thigh and the second pad over the sore area.

You should also lightly stretch the thigh muscles by gently pulling your heel to your buttock while standing on one leg.

Sore Calf Muscle

Calf muscles can become strained from sports and from overuse. Calf muscle pain is usually due to muscle cramps caused by lack of use and poor circulation.

To relieve pain and cramps in a calf muscle, place one electrode at the mid-calf area and a second electrode just behind the knee. The best treatment position is to lie on your back and rest your leg on a pillow to allow free ankle movement.

Ankle pump exercise: The ankle pump exercise consists of raising your toes toward your shin, then pointing them down. To promote circulation, perform the ankle pump exercise whenever possible, at least three to six times a day.

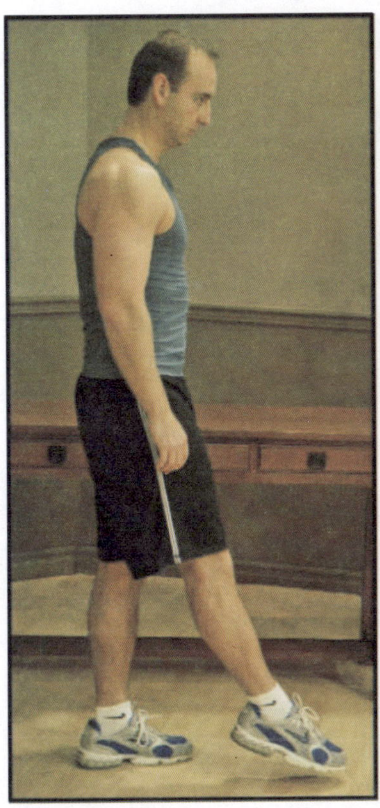

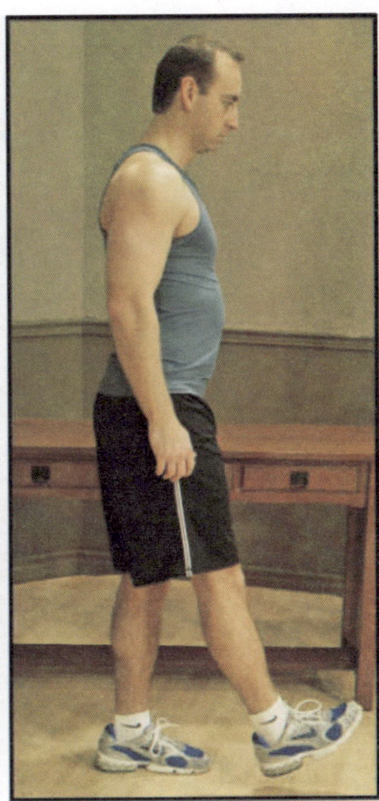

Hamstring Pain

Hamstring (the muscle at the back of your thigh) strain usually occurs from sports activities that involve running.

To treat the hamstring, place one electrode at mid-hamstring and the second electrode on the sore area. Rest the leg on a couple of pillows with the knee bent to allow the hamstring to be loose and free to move.

To stretch the hamstring, straighten your leg, place your heel on a counter and reach forward to touch your toes with one hand and then the other hand.

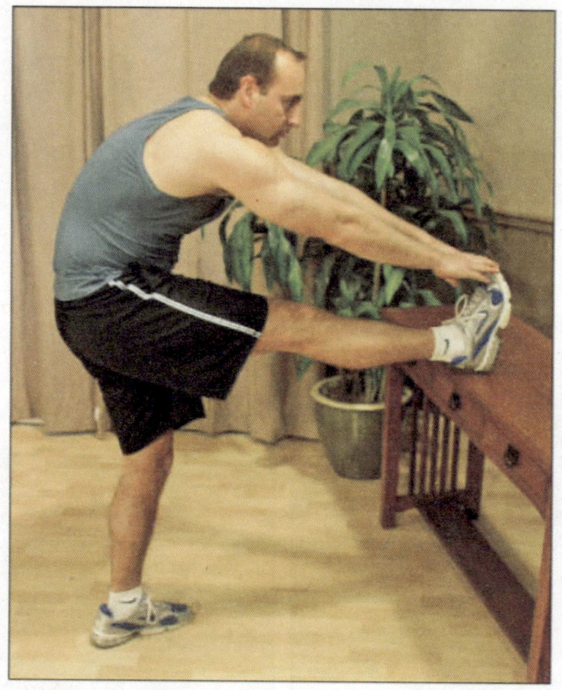

Shin Pain

Pain in the shin area can be caused by straining the shin muscles and from stress fractures in the shin bone. Lie on your back and place a couple of pillows under the knee, keeping the ankle relaxed. Place one electrode just below and to the right side of the knee and a second pad at the mid-shin.

You can stretch the shin muscle by gently sitting on the shin with your toes pointing down. Lower your weight slowly until you feel an adequate stretch.

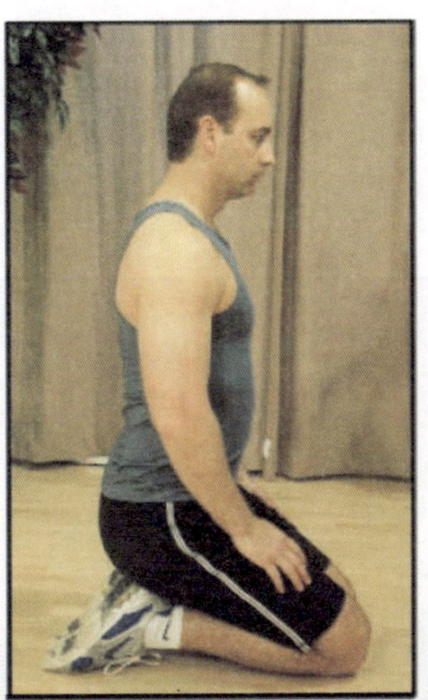

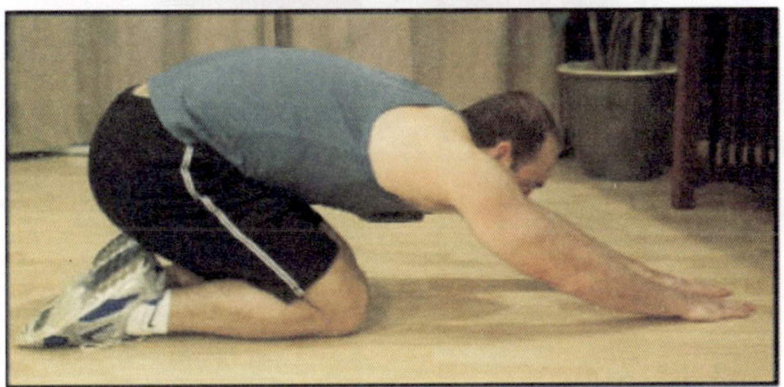

Ankle Pain

A sprained ankle can be very painful and can reoccur easily if the ligaments do not heal properly and if the different muscles that support the ankle are not balanced in tone.

To treat it, place one electrode on each side of the ankle.

Ankle exercise: To help reduce the inflammation, pump your ankle by moving your foot up and down when the foot is off the ground. Do the ankle pump exercise frequently throughout the day. To reset the muscle tone and balance, stand on the edge of a step and rise up on your toes and then lower your weight onto your heel. Perform this ankle-rocking exercise three to four sets each day, ten reps per set. Be sure to support yourself by holding onto something solid.

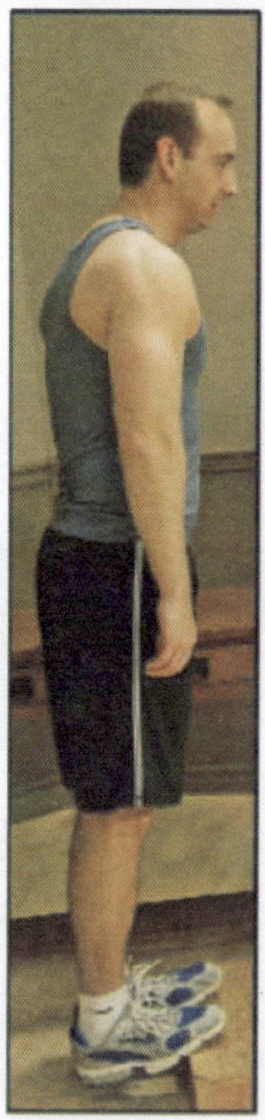

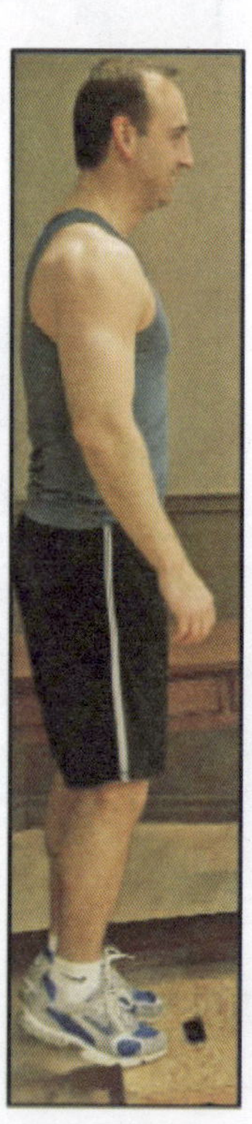

Foot Pain

Bad shoes are often the cause of foot pain. Prolonged standing in bad shoes can cause plantar fasciitis and heel spurs to form. Osteoarthritis, rheumatoid arthritis, gouty arthritis, poor circulation from diabetes and sciatica are all common causes of foot pain.

Specially designed Foot Relief Massage Pads can be used with *Dr. Ho's Muscle Massage System* for massaging the sole. Place the Foot Relief Pads on the floor a few inches apart from each other, then place your bare feet on the pads. Make sure that the pads are not touching each other; otherwise, the current will go directly through the pads and not into your feet. If you don't feel a massage sensation, wait for a few minutes – the sensation will come as your circulation gets going. Many people have lost some sensation in their feet from injuries and other ailments.

If you have a painful condition such as plantar fasciitis or heel spurs, massage your feet before bedtime and again in the morning before you put weight on them.

Menstrual Cramps

Many women experience lower abdominal cramps with each menstrual period. To relieve the muscle cramps and pain, place one electrode above another electrode on the midline area between the umbilicus and the pubic bone. If the cramping and pain are not completely gone after twenty to thirty minutes of treatment, you should then place the electrodes over your lower back muscles and upper tailbone area for further relief. Treating the lower back nerves often provides quick relief because they directly connect to organs in the lower abdomen.

Pain During Childbirth

We **do not** recommend using *Dr. Ho's Muscle Massage System* during pregnancy, because of the risk of premature labour. However, we highly recommend that you use it to ease some of the pain during childbirth, particularly if you are forgoing pain medication during the birthing process. Place the electrodes on your lower back and over the sacrum (upper tailbone area) during labour. You should ask your doctor and the hospital for permission to use *Dr. Ho's Muscle Massage System* prior to your delivery date. Many hospitals will provide you with a **TENS** device for the same purpose.

Facial Pain

Pain located behind the eyes, at the temple or over the forehead area is usually due to an irritated C1 and/or C2 nerve at the upper back part of the neck. For pain in these areas, treatment should be applied to the upper neck.

Pain in the jaw area just in front of the ear is usually due to **TMJ** (tight jaw) syndrome. More severe "shooting" pain in the facial area is probably related to a condition called *trigeminal neuralgia*. When a nerve in the face becomes inflamed, it can be very painful indeed.

Facial paralysis can also occur from a cerebral stroke or from a condition called Bell's palsy. With Bell's, the nerves become partially paralyzed for no known reason.

The treatment procedure for pain or muscle paralysis in the face using *Dr. Ho's Muscle Massage System* is the same. Place one electrode on the area just in front of the ear, put the second electrode on the forehead and stimulate the areas for about five minutes. Then move the electrode from the forehead onto the cheekbone and turn on the device for another five minutes. Lastly, move the electrode from the cheekbone onto the lower jaw and run the machine for another five minutes. You will have to hold the electrodes against your face because the pads will not stick to oily facial skin. Repeat this treatment frequently over the course of the day.

Paralysis Following Stroke

A cerebral stroke can cause paralysis or weakening in various muscle groups, depending on the areas of the brain that are affected. You may need to get a muscle chart, or a book with a muscle chart, to determine which muscle is not functioning and requires treatment. Once you've determined which muscle group needs to be stimulated, apply the electrodes accordingly. Place one electrode over the "belly," or midsection, of the muscle. Position the second electrode about three to six inches above or below the first. Stimulate each muscle group for at least twenty minutes at a time, three to six times per day every day until you reach maximum strength and recovery.

You will also need to work with your doctor and rehabilitation specialist to design a specific home-use exercise program to further your recovery. The sooner you begin your therapy, the better and more complete your recovery will be.

Herniated, Slipped Disc Therapy

Dr. Ho's Muscle Massage System can be used effectively for the treatment of herniated discs, protruded discs and degenerated disc or slipped disc syndrome.

The spinal disc is a circular ring of ligaments, with a jelly cushion centre, that sits between two vertebrae. When you have a degenerated disc, your doctor may inform you that your X-ray, **MRI** or **CAT** scan has revealed that you have a "herniated," "slipped" or "protruded" disc. All these terms imply the same findings: degeneration has caused the inner "jelly filling" to bulge against nerves, causing irritation that produces local and referred pain. In many cases, your doctor will recommend surgery to remove either part of or the entire disc. Before anyone with a degenerated disc rushes into surgery, there are a few considerations. The discovery of a protruded disc does not necessarily indicate that it is the cause of your pain. Many people have bulging discs without any symptoms at all. Conversely, many people have symptoms that mimic a disc herniation but no sign of actual herniation. The success rate for eliminating your symptoms with spinal surgery is very low. This surgery is also quite risky and should be utilized only as a last result when all other methods of treatment fail to give you adequate relief.

If you have a degenerated disc, it is very important to try *Dr. Ho's Muscle Massage System* on the muscles along your spine on a regular basis. All chronic spinal disorders involve tightly contracted muscles and scar tissue surrounding the discs. This chronic muscle tension will exert more pressure on your degenerated discs and cause more protrusion and pain. Chronic muscle tension will also restrict further joint movement and deprive the joint surfaces of the lubricating and nourishing synovial fluid. By treating yourself with *Dr. Ho's Muscle Massage* device, you'll be able to relax the muscles and relieve the pain. When the muscles are relaxed, you will remove pressure from the disc, allowing it to expand and hopefully reducing the protrusion. When the muscles are relaxed and lengthened, you can perform the appropriate passive joint movement exercises to restore maximum motion.

Treatment of Cervical Spondylitis

If you have cervical spondylitis, rest, medication and physiotherapy may take away most of your symptoms, but they do not treat the underlying cause. **NSAIDs** may help relieve some pain, but the relief will be temporary at best. For better results, try hot and cold therapies and an active exercise program. Exercises should include those that stretch and strengthen the neck and shoulders, as well as aerobic exercise to keep the body loose and fluid. Gentle massage, including **TENS** therapy, may help to not only limit your pain, but improve your posture as well, which will relieve some of the stress on your spine.

I also advise that you try the spine exercises detailed in the herniated disc section.

Implement a daily course of massage or **TENS** therapy, at least once in the morning and once before bed, being sure to treat the areas where your pain erupts. Touch the muscles along your spine until you find tender spots and place *Dr. Ho's Muscle Massage System* pads directly on them, using all four pads if needed for expansive treatment coverage.

Never place electrodes directly on the spine itself, but on those muscles that support it on either side.

Treatment for Arthritis and Spinal Stenosis

Osteoarthritis tends to show up in the wrist, hand, hip, knee and first toe. Rheumatoid arthritis can be severe and deforming depending on the age of onset and aggressiveness of the case. Spinal stenosis is arthritis of the spine itself. Whatever the type, the goal in treating arthritis is to involve therapies that accomplish the following:

1. *Reduce the inflammation.*
2. *Relieve the pain.*
3. *Maximize mobility.*
4. *Avoid reoccurrence.*
5. *Prevent joint erosion and deformity.*

Medical doctors, chiropractors, physiotherapists, massage therapists and acupuncturists all have effective treatment methods that can help with arthritis, including **TENS** therapy. Since arthritis is a chronic condition that requires long-term attention, daily self-care with an electrotherapy device is highly recommended by many health professionals.

While massage therapy will not cure arthritis, it can help reduce inflammation and pain. Combining massage therapy with the gentle passive joint exercises illustrated in this chapter can increase joint mobility and decrease the rate of joint degeneration. Studies have shown that massage therapy can also minimize dependency on medications such as **NSAIDs** and muscle relaxants for people with muscle, joint or nerve discomfort and pain.

For anyone suffering from spinal stenosis or other back pain, I highly recommend that you try the spine exercises detailed in the herniated disc section.

For people suffering from gouty arthritis, a metabolic disease that causes pain and swelling of the big toe and sometimes the knee, the best relief in addition to therapy is to avoid red meat and alcohol, which can encourage the buildup of metabolic by-products. For people whose condition cannot be relieved through diet, prescription medication can be very effective in keeping symptoms at bay, so consult with your doctor.

Treatment for Whiplash

In the past, whiplash injuries were often treated with immobilization techniques such as donning a cervical collar, a support device that limits neck movement. However, a joint that doesn't move properly will degenerate rapidly. For this reason the use of a cervical collar should be infrequent, if at all. Neck injuries respond best to gentle stretching and movement, while inactivity can and will cause them to become worse. Ice should be applied for the first twenty-four hours to reduce swelling, followed by gentle movement and stretching. Don't perform stretches to the point of pain – only gentle resistance. As soon as possible, you should begin aerobic activities such as walking or swimming. **TENS** is also enormously beneficial in restoring range of motion and aiding in tissue repair.

Mild to Moderate Neck Strain

Neck strain is usually caused by sleeping in an awkward position that puts tension on the muscles along the back of your neck. To loosen the muscles and reduce pain, stand in a hot shower for five minutes with the water running on the back of your neck. Then press your chin to your chest and hold for thirty seconds. Now turn your head from side to side ten times each (twenty times total). Doing this every morning should help heal mild strains. Massage and **TENS** treatment offer further relief and actually help to prevent common strain my keeping the neck muscles loose and toned. If you are prone to a stiff neck when you wake up, give your neck a **TENS** or massage treatment every morning and every night before bedtime to prevent neck muscle contraction.

Tips to Help Avoid Strain and Injury

These are general tips that people should be mindful of during the course of their daily routines. They can help prevent or limit the severity of "onset injuries" that can lead to serious problems later in life.

- *Always wear a seat belt when you are in a vehicle.*
- *Also in a vehicle, be sure your headrest is adjusted to the proper height to prevent the overextension of your neck during a sudden stop or impact.*
- *Never dive into a shallow pool, and be sure that young people are properly supervised when swimming and diving.*
- *Always wear the proper protective equipment for your sport, such as a helmet, shoulder pads and/or joint guards.*
- *Always ask for help when lifting a heavy object or performing difficult tasks.*
- *Commit yourself to good posture in all activities and during rest.*

Treating Migraine, Tension and Cervicogenic Headaches

There are many possible causes for headaches. Most types of headaches including migraines are related to excessive muscle tension at the upper neck area. Muscle tension at the back of the neck can cause headaches directly by irritating the nerve fibres that exit your neck and extend to your head. Tight neck muscles can decrease the blood circulation and cause pain in the head and neck area.

For most headaches, I've found that neck massage, exercise and relaxation techniques can produce quick relief without medication. If these methods will help your condition, you'll notice an improvement within the first half an hour. There's nothing to lose and it's easy to determine if your problem is related to your neck simply by trying massage techniques first, before you reach for the meds.

During my nineteen years of practice I've encountered only half a dozen patients whom I had to refer to neurologists because simple massage, exercise and relaxation techniques, or ergonomic and dietary advice, did not make a big difference. For roughly 99 percent of people I've treated, just restoring movement in the joints of the neck and upper back using *Dr. Ho's Muscle Massage System*, along with some lessons on posture and ergonomics, was enough to offer tremendous relief.

Use *Dr. Ho's Muscle Massage System* to relieve an existing headache or use it to treat yourself regularly to prevent headaches from occurring.

To treat your headache, lie comfortably on your back and support your neck with a rolled-up heavy towel, sponge roll or an orthopedic pillow. Your neck and head should feel supported but not cranked forward.

Place the electrodes at the top and back of the neck in the area just below the hairline, so that you can treat your C1 and C2 nerves. Place one electrode on each side of the spine (but not directly on the spine itself) to achieve balance. If you have tension or pain in the lower neck and upper shoulder, you should treat these areas as well since they can aggravate your headaches. Because *Dr. Ho's Muscle Massage System* comes with four electrode pads, you can easily treat all tense areas at the same time. As you massage your neck, try to focus on your breathing – close your eyes, relax and breathe in deeply through your nose to maximize your oxygen intake, and exhale slowly through your mouth. Once you get used to this technique, try pushing out your abdomen as you inhale (as if your belly is filling with air) and bringing it in slowly as you exhale. This method can help you to relax faster and more completely.

To give yourself treatment when you feel a headache coming on, apply pressure to the top part of the back of your neck with your thumb and hold for ten seconds. Repeat as needed. As a regular exercise to restore normal motion in your neck, simply rotate your neck from side to side within your comfort range. Turn your neck ten times each side every thirty minutes. Do this daily until your neck can move in a full and comfortable range of motion.

A Word About Medications

Medication can be helpful when used correctly, but too often meds are expected to be magical cures for pain, which is not the case. Pain medication can indeed provide some temporary relief of pain, which can be highly positive when other methods fail. It can be particularly useful during the first stages of an injury when the reduction of inflammation will facilitate normal movement so that the body can heal itself.

But pain medication should not be your first line of defense whenever you suffer a pain episode. There are many other treatment options to consider that are just as (and often more) effective than medication. For example, some people find that non-prescription commercial analgesics, such as **BENGAY**, offer quicker pain relief when applied directly to sore or injured areas than pills can provide. Also worth noting is that at least one clinical study holds that commercial heat wraps, such as ThermaCare, are more effective in relieving muscle pain than over-the-counter pain medication.

When your condition warrants medication, I still suggest that you use it in conjunction with other treatments: massage therapy such as TENS; stretching techniques from the ones I've outlined here to more advanced routines like yoga; chiropractic, osteopathic and/or acupuncture treatments where indicated; and always a regular routine of exercises. All of these involve improving your body and your health, which will offer you far greater and more lasting relief than medication alone.

Medication Choices

For general pain conditions, your doctor may prescribe either an over-the-counter drug or a prescription. Here are some common choices:

- **Non-steroidal anti-inflammatory drugs** *(NSAIDs): including Aspirin, ibuprofen (Advil, Motrin and others) and naproxen (Aleve), these can temporarily relieve pain and reduce inflammation, but many can cause stomach irritation, even bleeding. Any of them can have a negative interaction with other medications, so check with your doctor if you take anything else. A new breed of NSAIDs are called COX II inhibitors, and they include celecoxib (Celebrex) and rofecoxib (Vioxx), which may be less likely than other NSAIDs to cause stomach irritation. A word of caution, however: COX II inhibitor drugs are typically not incorporated in the treatment of many people because they may increase the risk of heart attack, even in people under age sixty, so talk to your doctor.*

- **Acetaminophen** *(Tylenol): this drug has less interaction problems than most other pain medications, but many people find its relief inadequate. Dosage also requires that you take it every four hours that you're in pain, which can lead to headaches* *associated with overexposure to pain meds. Acetaminophen has also been shown to have very negative effects on some people who drink alcohol or are fasting.*

- **Muscle relaxants**: *these are used to treat severe neck pain and spasm, but they can make a person feel "spacey" and unable to concentrate. It is advisable to refrain from operating vehicles or other heavy machinery while taking muscle relaxants. They can also cause other unpleasant side effects such as constipation.*

- **Narcotic (prescription) pain relievers**: *these include a wide array of choices, from Vicodin to codeine, but should be used for a short term only because all can be highly addictive and cause many unwanted side effects, such as an inability to concentrate, lethargy and constipation. None should be mixed with alcohol. Any of the medications described here, as well as others, can produce both short-term and long-term side effects that range from mildly annoying to very dangerous. So please don't get into the habit of taking medication simply because you were offered a prescription. Always explore other methods to treat pain conditions first, and leave medication as your second-to-last choice, just ahead of surgery. And always remember not to overdo any medication, as some can cause a "rebound" effect that will invite the very pain you're trying to get rid of.*

Consider all four pillars of health when you think of the overall picture of your well-being: take care of your body through exercise, proper diet and holistic therapies, and take care of your heart and soul by seeking out positive environments and limiting negative ones. If you can adhere to these concepts for an eight-week test period, I can all but guarantee that you'll emerge a changed person who will never go back to your old habits again. Reading this book was your first step on the path to better health and vitality, and it is my greatest hope that your journey will be rewarding beyond measure. You have my best wishes and support in this and in all the positive changes you will make in your life. Good luck!

Neck Traction Therapy

Traction Therapy, the gentle lengthwise stretching of the spine, has been used for centuries to alleviate the pain associated with spinal nerve compression disorders. In fact, there is documentation that axial traction was used by the ancient Egyptians to treat spinal dislocation as far back as 3000 BC. Modern traction therapies came into widespread use in the early 1930s, and their many forms and applications have received the gamut of conclusions, from quite effective to not at all, or even injurious. What has become key to effective traction therapy is its controlled use-specifically, statistics support that traction methodologies are most effective and safest when the patient is allowed to adjust and limit the intensity used to stretch the spine and its associated tissues, which both eliminates risk of over-force injury and allows immediate relief and long-term recovery. When used regularly and appropriately, studies have shown that fully 25% of patients who were relegated to the final desperate treatment of surgery to relieve compression-related disorders, including herniated discs, degenerated facet joints and pinched nerves, were able to forego surgery altogether. Furthermore, numerous research studies, as well as my own clinical observations, show that over the long term, therapeutic electrical stimulation combined with patient-controlled traction is more effective than surgery, as well as safer, non-invasive and undisruptive to normal living-all at a fraction of the cost and recuperation time.

As we age, gravity, overuse and poor posture can invite compression or dislocation of the vertebrae in the upper spine, and can cause it to lose its natural cervical lordosis, or backward curvature. Diagnostic imaging often reveals that patients with neck, head and upper back and limb pain have cervical spines that have straightened over time, or even begun to list to one side. Because it receives no real rest during waking hours as it balances the 10+ pound orb of the head, the cervical spine and its joints and discs are especially vulnerable to compression disorders. This slow degeneration can cause serious pain, not only in the neck itself, but in any area served by the cervical spine's root system, such as the head and those associated with the nerve structure known as the brachial plexus, including the upper and lateral back muscles, upper chest, shoulders, forearms, elbows, hands and fingers. Pressure on the nerve roots of the spinal vertebrae, whether from degenerative disc disease, herniated discs or a narrowing within the spine called spinal stenosis, will commonly refer pain to the areas of the upper body served by the impacted nerves, causing burning, aching, weakness and/or numbness, a condition known medically as cervical radiculopathy.

Traction therapy offers relief and correction by gently stretching the muscles along the spine and decompressing the spinal discs that separate the vertebrae, releasing the pressure on the roots that serve the lateral, posterior and medial cords, whose nerves branch through the shoulders, arms and into the hands. This anatomical relationship is why alleviating pressure on the neck can restore circulation and alleviate pain in such far-away locations as the elbow, wrist or fingers.

In my 20 years of clinical practice, I've found traction therapy to be extremely beneficial to patients suffering from cervical spine-related pain syndromes, including headaches and neck, shoulder and trapezius (where the lower neck meets the upper back) muscle stiffness and pain, as well as aching, numbness and weakness in the upper limbs. Because most head and upper body pain syndromes involve the nerves that exit the cervical spine, treatment at the source is always the first, and usually most effective, course of treatment.

Why do so many people suffer from neck tension-related disorders?

Let's be honest-life is stressful, both physically and emotionally. If you've ever had someone rub your neck and shoulders, you've probably become immediately aware of how tense those areas are, even if you weren't cognizant of it before you were touched. That's not typically true of other areas, such as your arms or legs. This is because the spine is the unfortunate repository of the long list of everyday stresses and abuses, from the ergonomic stress of a poor working environment, to the slumping you do in front of the TV, to the anger you must silently absorb dealing with a rigid boss, a crying child or those drivers who ride your bumper on the highway. Northern Americans typically compound the effects of these stressors by engaging in too little physical activity, and over time the vulnerable areas, particularly the neck, absorb the abuse. Added to the natural processes of aging, the discs in the cervical spine degenerate and weaken. As the discs become increasingly vulnerable to pressure, less force is required to cause a degenerated disc to become herniated, or to "slip," wherein the outside layer of the disc ruptures and the inner gel extrudes and presses against the adjacent nerve roots. As a result, middle-aged adults-whose intervertebral cushioning diminishes with time-are more susceptible to herniated discs. Once rupture occurs, the irritation of disc against disc can invite bony spurs to develop near the nerve roots, which can induce agonizing pain, numbness and weakness in the neck, shoulders and back. Warning symptoms include (1) sore neck and shoulder muscles; (2) numbness or poor circulation in the hands and/or head; (3) lack of energy; and (4) pain behind the eyes and/or around the temples. Left untreated, common and often debilitating syndromes such as migraines, tension headaches, carpal tunnel syndrome, arthritis, tendonitis, bursitis, and chronic neck pain can develop and adversely affect every aspect of one's life. Vast research-including clinical studies in peer-reviewed medical literature and evidence-based guidelines from public health agencies, as well as my own empirical experience with patients-verifies that the most curative treatment for chronic cervical spine compression syndromes is daily therapy that includes active movement to keep spinal joints flushed and lubricated, methods to improve blood flow such as massage or electrical stimulation (TENS), and the gentle passive stretching involved in traction.

Beyond simple stretching, appropriate cervical traction has proven to improve, even restore, the natural curvature of the cervical spine in as few as 8-10 weeks, and the improvements were determined to remain with simple maintenance therapy. Clinical trials also confirm that a combined therapy of traction, electrical stimulation and exercise promote immediate and measurable improvement in cervical radiculopathy patients' grip strength and facility, owing, researchers believe, to increased blood flow to and from the cervical nerve roots serving the arms and hands.

Chronic tension and migraine headaches

As discussed in Chapter Four: Migraine and Tension Headache, almost all headaches not owing to a pathogenic cause can be effectively managed and oftentimes prevented entirely through a combination treatment program of massage therapy, exercise, good posture practices and relaxation/breathing exercises. Also paramount in treating and preventing tension and/or compression-related headaches is gentle neck traction to relieve muscle tension in the upper neck, where the nerves exit and branch into the head. When the neck muscles experience stress, whether physical, emotional or both, they tighten and cause a stiff, sore neck. The tension and inflammation, though invisible to the eye, irritate the uppermost cervical nerves, and cause the majority of sufferers' headaches.

When asked, an interesting number of people tell me that either they have little stress in their lives, or that they're able to handle it adequately. If you find parts of your body, such as your neck, head or upper, mid- or low-back sore without a specific cause (such as overexerting yourself on the tennis court or falling down stairs), then you probably haven't conquered stress as effectively as you think. For 99.9% of us, stress isn't a one-time event, but a cumulative cycle of absorbing, ignoring and then sometimes overreacting to a "trigger event" (such as discovering someone left an empty milk carton in the fridge or being trapped behind a bank customer who wants to deposit $100 in loose change). Add to your mental taxation the constant physical stress, from the prosaic, such as sitting at the office desk all day or performing repetitive activities, to the dramatic, like suffering whiplash in an accident, and that's a fine recipe for spinal and muscular strain, which may or may not show its damage immediately.

Since quitting your job, duties and activities isn't an option, it's important to learn how to prevent and treat pain conditions before they become chronic or, if they've already progressed to that point, find ways to abate-even cure-them over time. I have treated countless patients suffering from chronic headaches, most of whom have been prescribed myriad medications to mask the symptoms, but because headaches are so difficult to medically diagnose ("tension" is a vague term at best, and many MDs aren't trained in stress relief), the root causes are often left undiscovered. Thus, despite an abundance of medication, the headaches persist. As a headache specialist, I've found that a combination of neck traction, chiropractic spinal manipulation, massage and/or electrical stimulation therapy, neck and shoulder exercises, and improved posture can be incredibly effective in preventing the reoccurrence of migraines and tension headaches. More good news is that properly and consistently applied home treatment, even without concurrent chiropractic care, also provides remarkable results, enabling chronic headache sufferers to receive reliable, affordable care in the privacy and convenience of their own homes.

To illustrate the efficacy of at-home therapy, allow me to share the experience of one of my patients.

The migraine headache patient

When she first came to my office, Kim was a forty year-old nurse who had spent the previous 12 years working in a hospital helping others. For more than 10 of those years she'd suffered debilitating migraines, and had reached a point where her headaches forced her to miss work. Even with time off, her headaches persisted as often as 4-5 days a week, and she was constantly taking painkillers and migraine medications to provide temporary relief just to get through the day. By the time she came to my clinic, she was resigned to the fact that she would live the rest of her life in pain and dependent upon medication. Kim had been to many specialists and received numerous X-rays, CAT scans, MRIs and blood tests, none of which pinpointed a direct cause of her headaches.

As is typical of migraines, Kim's headaches produced very intense pain in one temple and horrible throbbing behind the adjacent eye. Noise and bright light aggravated her misery and she often experienced nausea and vomiting. Her other symptoms included numbness in her hands, and soreness and stiffness in her neck and shoulder muscles. X-rays revealed a spine compressed by years of poor posture and the early signs of disc and joint degeneration. Her history as a nurse included constantly lifting and assisting patients, and over time these duties created chronic tension and inflammation in her neck muscles, which were in turn irritating the upper cervical nerves and causing her migraines.

Our treatment objective was to reduce her neck and shoulder muscle tension, thereby limiting irritation to the affected nerves.

I recommended that she use the DR-HO'S® Muscle Massage System on her upper neck three times a day for eight weeks, with additional treatments whenever she felt the onset of a headache. Using the massage system relieved her muscle tension, reduced the pain in her neck and shoulders, increased the circulation to her head, and improved the range of motion in her neck. This was a vital first step in her ability to reclaim her health. I also recommended that she engage in daily neck traction to release pressure from her cervical vertebrae and restore good posture. Every day after work Kim would apply 20 minutes of gentle traction using the DR-HO'S® Neck Comforter™ to release the stress from her neck muscles, and then again before she went to bed.

After about two weeks of combined at-home electrical stimulation and neck traction, Kim reported amazing results. Her headaches had decreased dramatically from 4-5 headaches every week to only 1-2 headaches for the entire two-week therapy period. Whenever Kim felt the onset of a headache, she immediately applied electrical massage for instant relief, followed by gentle neck traction. During the following month of treatment, Kim reported only one mild headache. She was off pain medication and reported feeling revitalized, energetic and optimistic for the first time in eight years. She also reported that it was not just she who felt relieved-her family, coworkers and friends were also thrilled to have her back to her wonderful, happy self. To protect her health and energy, Kim maintains regular traction and massage therapy to keep her neck and shoulder muscles relaxed, and to prevent future headaches from occurring.

The carpal tunnel patient

While it may seem understandable that neck traction treatment is beneficial to people suffering from headaches, people are often surprised to learn that neck traction, in addition to electrical stimulation, is an extremely effective treatment for the agonizing pain in the hands, fingers and forearms caused by carpal tunnel syndrome. CTS afflicts many whose jobs or hobbies involve improper or overuse of the hands and/or fingers, including assembly line tasks, sports, working with certain substances or tools, and, of course, the most heinous of all culprits, working at a computer.

Typical treatment for CTS involves immobilizing the affected wrist with a splint or removable cast, which offers relief because the nerves are allowed to calm, but once activity resumes the pain returns. The last ditch effort is usually surgery to widen the cramped carpal tunnel, which in most cases makes about as much sense as improving your golf game by widening the hole instead of working on your swing. After all, the nerves' impingement isn't caused because the carpal tunnel is shrinking, but rather because the nerves are inflamed and pressing against the passage.

Like most upper-body repetitive stress disorders, CTS occurs when nerves in your lower neck and/or upper back are inflamed or pinched. These nerves serve the bundles and branches of the brachial plexus, which traverses your collarbone to your shoulders and then down your arms in different distributions. These branches include the median and ulnar nerves, which pass through the tiny hard "tunnel" at the base of your palm where it meets your wrist, giving sensation to your fingers and thumb.

If the C7 cervical nerve in the lower neck/upper back is irritated, inflammation and swelling of the median and/or ulnar nerves can cause either or both to become impinged within the bony carpal tunnel, making movement of the hands and fingers invite pain, burning, tingling, weakness, numbness, iciness and/or clumsiness.

This anatomical arrangement is why effective treatment for carpal tunnel syndrome should start with the malady's origins-the cervical vertebrae and its nerve roots-rather than simply the site of pain; this therapy applies to a host of other overuse injuries as well, including lateral epicondylitis (tennis elbow), medial epicondylitis (golfer's elbow), rotator cuff tendonitis, tendosynovitis of the finger, thoracic outlet syndrome, and others. For more on the cause and treatment of these problems, please refer to Chapter Three: Identifying the Problem.

In my experience, it is always superior to treat the problem first, and let the symptoms subside as health improves-only then can you promote the properties of healing pain instead of simply masking it.

For example, let's review the case of one of my CTS patients:

Jennifer, a thirty-one year-old customer service representative, spent 6-8 hours at her computer station every workday. Over time she developed repetitive strain injury in her wrist and neck, causing pain so severe she could barely lift the affected arm, and was suffering constant headaches. She had no choice but to take sick leave from her job so she could seek out different specialists, all of whom told her that she had carpal tunnel syndrome. The solution they suggested was surgery to widen the carpal tunnel, followed by a recovery period of 6-8 months. When asked if her headaches had anything to do with the pain in her wrist and arm, she was told that there was no relation between the two. Out of sheer desperation, she booked a date for surgery.

Through pure coincidence, I met Jennifer on an airplane and she idly mentioned her upcoming surgery. I inquired about her symptoms and found her condition similar to many of my patients'. I explained that her condition was very common and that the root of the problem was not in her wrist, but in her neck, and suggested that she try a course of neck traction and electrical stimulation therapy before resorting to surgery.

Although she was admittedly skeptical, Jennifer began a therapy program using DR-HO'S® Muscle Massage System to treat her neck, shoulders, and wrists, combined with 20-minute neck traction sessions, 3 times a day. After only one month her improvement was so substantial that she not only cancelled her surgery, she also returned to work. The simple mechanism of gently stretching and relaxing her neck removed the constant irritation from her cervical nerves and relieved her CTS, and the pain and duration of her headaches decreased significantly as well.

With continued therapy, Jennifer reported that she no longer experienced the sharp, shooting pains in her wrist and forearm and had regained sensation in her fingertips. Since her job continues to pose the same demands, she now prevents recurrence of her problems by following a maintenance program using the DR-HO'S® Muscle Massage System in conjunction with the DR-HO'S® Neck Comforter™ traction unit to alleviate pressure and prevent tension buildup. Both Jennifer and her family were pleased to find this alternative to surgery, and as my patients will attest, neck traction is a pleasant, non-invasive way not only to treat present maladies, but also to prevent future pain episodes altogether.

At-home neck traction therapy

Research indicates that 1 in 10 North Americans suffers from non-traumatic (not related to direct force or accident) neck disorders. The pain source may involve muscles, ligaments, bones or all of these, but the root causes are typically improper mechanical use of the neck and/or degenerative processes that cause compression of neural structures, inflammation and muscular spasm.

The key to effective traction therapy for cervical spine-related disorders is patient-controlled tension (the amount of pressure used to separate the spinal discs) and its regular use over the long term, not only to help solve pain problems but to prevent their recurrence. The DR-HO'S® Neck Comforter™ traction unit is designed to use patient-controlled inflation, allowing for the gradual, gentle adjustment of the stretch applied to the neck muscles and spine, assuring that pressure never overextends or injures the fragile anatomy of cervical structures.

When inflated, The Neck Comforter™ utilizes passive traction and neutral alignment to gently lift the weight of your head off your neck, promoting the relaxation and safe stretching of muscles and spinal discs, and increasing nerve and blood circulation throughout the neck, head and upper limbs. The unit supports the natural curve (lordosis) of the cervical spine and removes pressure from cervical discs. And unlike some ill-conceived strap traction devices of the past, The Neck Comforter™ will not cause or aggravate temporomandibular joint conditions (TMJ). In only 20 minutes, The Neck Comforter™ helps relieve pain and promote healing of the following conditions:

- Herniated and/or compressed discs
- Degenerated facet joints
- Muscular spasm
- Headaches
- Pinched nerves
- Tension and stiffness in the neck and shoulders
- Poor blood and lymphatic circulation
- Improper posture
- Stress

Before Hernia & After Traction Therapy

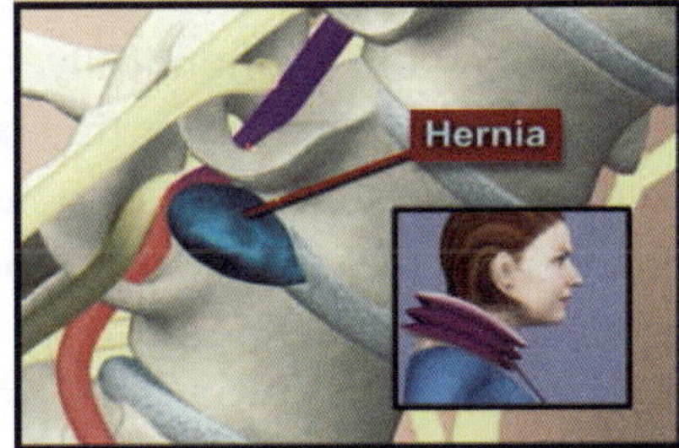

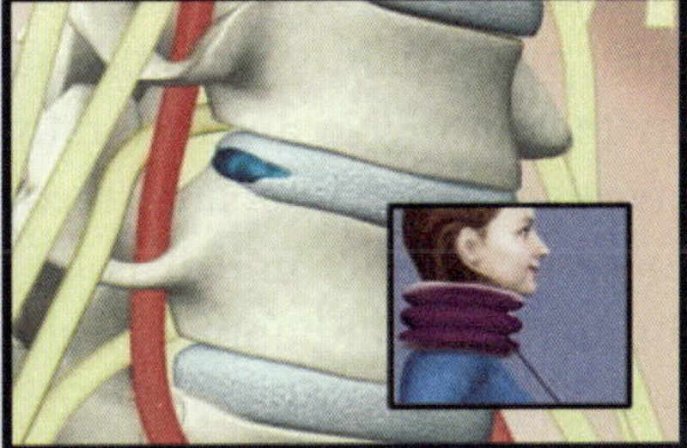

Before Degenerated Joint & After Traction Therapy

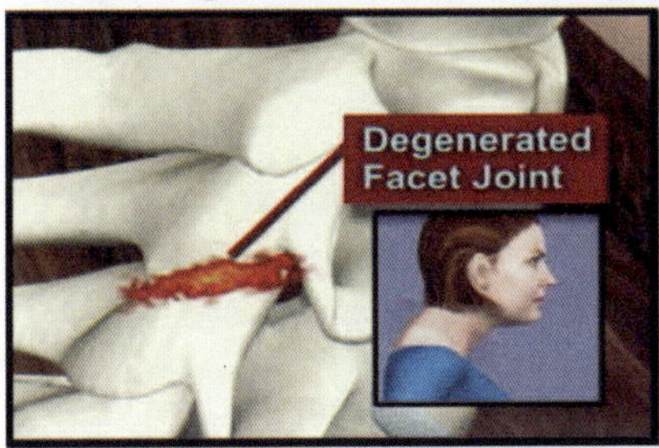

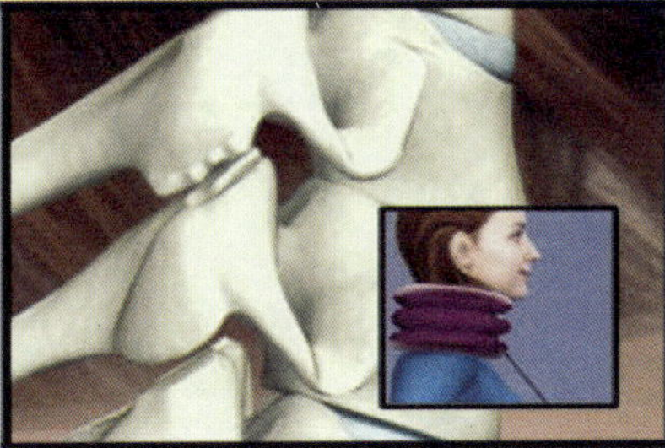

Before Traction Therapy & After Traction Therapy

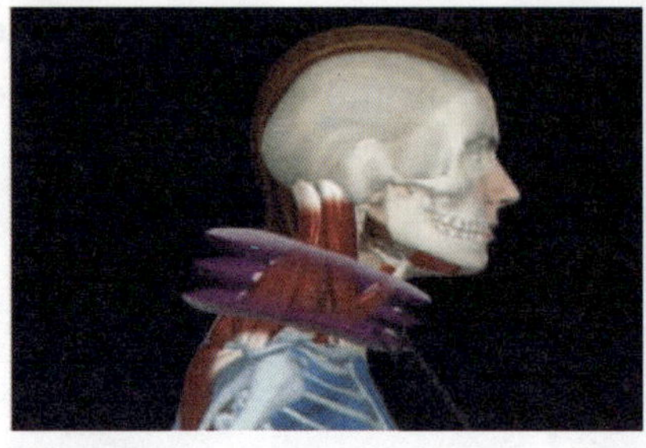

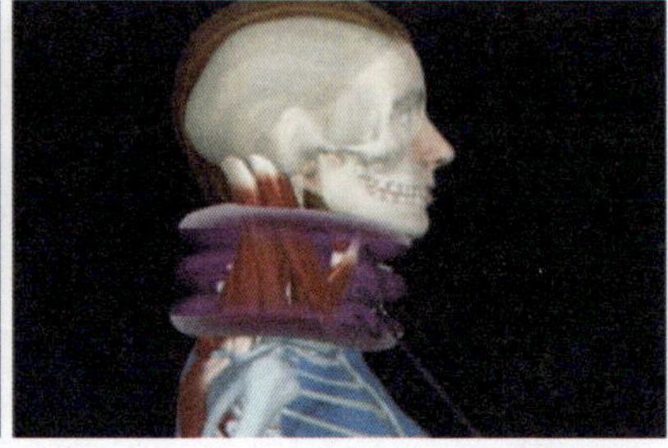

It has always been my position that treatment of the cause of disease and dysfunction is more beneficial and effective than addressing only the associated symptoms. By treating the root of the problem, ongoing suffering and dependency on painkillers can be greatly reduced or even eliminated entirely. During my two decades of clinical practice, I have learned that a combination of traction and massage can help people manage, and sometimes cure, many pain syndromes safely, quickly and economically. I invite you to give this restorative therapy a try before resorting to invasive, expensive and recovery-intensive solutions such as surgery-you may find it is all you need to feel better now and throughout your happier, healthier life ahead.

Patient Testimonials

When I developed the prototype for *Dr. Ho's Muscle Massage System*, my initial goal was to use it on the patients at my clinic. The typical response was: "Wow! I feel so much better. Can I buy one of these machines somewhere? Can I rent it over the weekend?" Almost immediately, my clinic had hundreds of people offering to buy the device. I was hesitant about branching out from my very busy (and time-consuming) chiropractic practice but people made countless phone calls to my office, eagerly offering deposits for the manufacture of an identical TENS product that they could use at home. It was their persistence that motivated me to mass-produce *Dr. Ho's Muscle Massage System*.

Dr. Ho's Muscle Massage System rapidly became the best-selling product on the Canadian Shopping Channel two years in a row, and shortly thereafter it enjoyed great success across the US market. Most importantly, through sales of the device I was able to positively change many people's lives, far more than I would have otherwise. I'm very happy to say that *Dr. Ho's Muscle Massage System* has enabled me to help a large and growing segment of the population – from those suffering from simple everyday stress and muscle tension, to those recovering from car accidents, to those suffering from everything from arthritis to fibromyalgia. Moreover, in a study conducted by an automotive parts manufacturing facility, the use of *Dr. Ho's Muscle Massage System* by its workers has helped to reduce health costs to the company while decreasing sick leaves due to joint pain and repetitive strain to the neck, shoulders, lower back and other areas. This finding pleases me beyond words.

TENS therapy is perhaps the most exciting discovery in pain treatment in the past three decades. Only twenty minutes is long enough to provide remarkable relief from any acute or chronically painful condition, and repeated use of *Dr. Ho's Muscle Massage System* offers long-term relief and, in many cases, full recovery. Because *Dr. Ho's Muscle Massage System* is a safe and drugless solution, you can use it as often as you want without worrying about negative side effects; it has met or exceeded all international safety and effectiveness standards. And though it is a very powerful device, my team and I designed it to require only two **AAA** batteries and to be small enough (about the size of a deck of cards) to take anywhere: work, travel, the basketball court or the baseball diamond, and of course to your home where you relax after a stressful day. It offers relief for over twenty different common conditions:

- *headaches*
- *neck pain*
- *shoulder tension*
- *rotator cuff tendinitis*
- *tennis elbow*
- *golfer's elbow*
- *carpal tunnel syndrome*
- *hand pain*
- *mid-back pain*

- *lower back pain*
- *hip pain*
- *sciatica*
- *groin pain*
- *knee pain*
- *thigh and hamstring pulls*
- *calf muscle pulls*
- *poor circulation*
- *ankle sprains*
- *plantar fasciitis and heel spur*
- *abdominal muscle pain*
- *menstrual tension*
- *jaw pain*
- *trigeminal neuralgia*
- *stiffness, joint inflammation and pain due to joint degeneration from osteoarthritis, gouty arthritis, rheumatoid arthritis or other injuries*
- *pain from diseases associated with muscle tension and poor circulation*

Pain from all these maladies can be reduced and even eliminated by simply increasing blood and nerve circulation and relaxing tense muscles. But the many hundreds of letters that I receive from happy users of the device can applaud its virtues far more eloquently than I, so please let me share with you just a few:

DEAR DR. HO:

I once had chronic lower back pain, but recently I have been using your system at least twice a day and I feel great! It is a drastic improvement on seeking similar treatment from appointments with chiropractors – at a great deal of expense and time. It's so great to be able to use your system any time and virtually anywhere, even at work (where it's very easy to conceal underneath my clothing).

I highly recommend your system to anyone experiencing any kind of muscular pain or simply looking for some relaxation. It puts me to sleep! I also use it on my Achilles tendon that I tore, and am now able to walk much better.

I will continue to use your muscle massage system forever. Dr. Ho, thank you for making my life better and pain-free!

– Janet Gurney; Oldsmar, Florida

DEAR DR. HO:

I have been suffering from chronic upper shoulder blade and neck pain for about two years. I began using the Dr. Ho unit in January, on average of four to five times per week, usually at bedtime. I put it on the affected area for about twenty minutes and I am able to go to sleep with decreased pain. Prior to using Dr. Ho I was reliant on painkillers. Now I just use Dr. Ho and don't need to take any pills. Thank you for a great product!

– Marie Tomasko; Wayne, New Jersey

DEAR DR. HO:

As the result of a car accident, for the past nine years I have suffered from severe neck and back pain. Doctors have prescribed me strong painkillers and muscle relaxants but they only mask the pain. A month ago my father, who is a doctor, purchased Dr Ho's Muscle Massage System for me. From the first twenty-minute session I noticed a bigger difference than years of taking pills. The day after I received Dr Ho's Muscle Massage System I threw away all of my medication. My neck and back are now virtually pain-free, and I feel as though I have been given a new lease on life. This product is simple to use and incredibly effective! Thank you!

— David Cooper; London, England

DEAR DR. HO:

I used to get bad neck pain for years, but now that I have tried Dr Ho's Muscle Massage System it has totally gone away! I love how the massage makes me feel, and it instantly takes away any neck pain I happen to have. I would recommend this system to anybody, whether or not they have problems or injuries — it feels so relaxing! Thanks a lot, Dr. Ho!

— Justin Versteeg; Burnaby, British Columbia

DEAR DR. HO:

I have suffered from migraine headaches and fibromyalgia for years. I purchased your muscle massager a few months ago and it has made a tremendous difference in my life. I sit at a computer all day and get terrible neck and shoulder pain. Since using Dr Ho's Muscle Massage System I have been able to cut back on the number of pain pills and muscle relaxants I was taking each day. I actually use the massager while at my desk at work! It's wonderful – no longer do I suffer while doing my job. My quality of life has improved dramatically since I bought the massager! Thank you – I wish I had had it years ago!

– Pat Kissel; Hanover Park, Illinois

DEAR DR. HO:

I have suffered from headaches and neck tension for over twenty years. I've tried physiotherapy and chiropractic therapy, and have taken many, many pain pills and relaxants. I obtained relief from the first time I used Dr Ho's Muscle Massage System. I initially bought a professional TENS unit for over $400 and it did not have the features that your device has. I love the relaxing waves of massage. I have passed it throughout my family and even took it to work and let ten co-workers try it. Everyone loved it!

Thanks so much for inventing a product that I can use so often and so easily. I bought it off the Home Shopping Network and figured if I didn't like it I would send it back, but NO WAY*! It's mine to keep! I have one suggestion: a small clip so I can secure it to my jeans. Everything else is great!*

– Kathy Padulese; Sewell, New Jersey

Note from Dr. Ho: Because of helpful feedback from users like Kathy, the system now has a convenient clip so that it can hook onto any pant, skirt or pocket.

DEAR DR. HO:

I suffered a severe neck injury, torticollis, in 1967. The problem was compounded by a car accident in 1975. In essence, I have had thirty-four years of chronic neck pain – some days agonizing, other days just sore. Over the last few years, because of deterioration in my cervical spine, the pain has required ice packs and frequent painkillers including 222's. Today I tried your machine: after twenty minutes on my trapezius muscles and ten minutes on the back of my neck (using all three programs), I've found the relief to be amazing! I can't believe how relaxed my neck is. I'm especially impressed with the ease of use and the amount of power in something small enough to fit into my pocket. Now I'll take my personal masseuse everywhere. Thanks for a pain relief machine that really works!

– Mike Mandel; Toronto, Ontario

DEAR DR. HO:

I just had my forty-first birthday. I've had fibromyalgia for fourteen years. I've tried exercises, physiotherapy, heating pads and painkillers – both over-the-counter and prescription. Nothing has helped. I ordered Dr Ho's Muscle Massage System hoping it would help my migraine headaches, and it did, but I also noticed a huge difference in my fibromyalgia. It was better for the first time in fourteen years!

Within three weeks of using it for the first time, I was sleeping at night without any pain. I could play with my children and be a real mom again. This may sound odd, but I would have to say that it changed not only my life, but my children's also: they got their mom back. Recently, my nine-year-old daughter was having a flare-up of her juvenile rheumatoid arthritis, and I let her use the Massage System on the gentle setting of low. In the words of a child, she said it helped the pain and made her feel better. I am ordering two more: one more for our family and one for my dad. Thank you, it's made a huge change in our family.

– Kathy Waldrup; Lilburn, Georgia

DEAR DR. HO:

Where to start? I suffer from neck and knee pain but worst of all is the tennis elbow: I have been fighting with pain on and off for about five years. When I saw the show on the Home Shopping Network for Dr Ho's Muscle Massage System, I figured it would be worth a shot. The first time I used the Massage System it felt a little strange, but about five minutes after I was finished I noticed I didn't have any pain in my elbow. Now when I get home from work, instead of reaching for the Tylenol I reach for my massager, which in most cases takes care of the problem immediately and feels great in the process. Thank you Dr. Ho, you're a lifesaver!!

– Shawn Haley; Baldwin Park, California

DEAR DR. HO:

I damaged my sciatic nerve last November, resulting in a complete loss of the use of my right leg and continuous extreme pain from muscle spasms. I ordered Dr Ho's Muscle Massage System in December from the Home Shopping Network. It has been a wonderful tool to relax the muscles from spasms and help my sciatic nerve to heal. I've had such wonderful results that my mother has borrowed it to help ease the pain in her middle back. It's worth every penny! I am so glad that I bought it. I also like the handy carrying case – it helps to keep my unit in good working condition. Thanks so much.

– Paulette Heller; Louisville, Kentucky

DEAR DR. HO:

Please let me tell you how much your Muscle Massage System has helped me. I have had a problem with my lower back/left hip for almost eleven years. I have been to physiotherapy, which helped a lot but I was still never completely pain-free and it became too expensive and time-consuming to keep up after six months. I was given Daypro and Darvocet and exercises to do at home between weekly visits. I had resigned myself to the fact that I was going to have this problem forever. Sometimes I had a very hard time walking because of the incredible pain, but nothing ever showed up in X-rays so it was difficult to prove that I had it.

I ordered your system two weeks ago, and I was on vacation when it arrived so I could immediately use it as often as I wanted. I can't believe it but now I am almost PAIN-FREE!!!!!!!!! Thank you so much for putting your invention on the market.

Tonight I saw your system again on the Home Shopping Network with extra-large pads. I called the HSN *to see about getting them but I was told they were no longer available. Please let me know how to order the larger pads. Thanks again for your great product.*

– Sandra Moody; Hutchins, Texas

*Note from Dr. Ho: For all of you who want to order the larger FlexTone pads, you can do so by simply calling us toll-free at 1-877-374-6669 (1-877-*DR HO NOW*). Or visit our Web site at* **www.drhonow.com**.

DEAR DR. HO:

In May 2001 a physiotherapist diagnosed my recent 40 percent reduction in strength as "tennis elbow," caused from ten-pin bowling over the winter season. The pain began in January and steadily increased as each week passed. I started treatment with my Dr. Ho on June 14, using the machine for twenty-minute sessions three to five times each day. Within a week I started to notice the pain was going away and the strength in my arm was increasing. It has been almost a month now and I have experienced a major improvement in mobility and considerably less pain in my arm when golfing or typing for several hours a day. I find this product extremely easy to use, even while walking or riding. With a little scotch tape to hold the pads in place, it is truly mobile! Thank you Dr. Ho for giving me the ability to rebound from this injury and play the sports that I love.

– Janice Love; Mississauga, Ontario

DEAR DR. HO:

One morning I woke up with such extreme pain in my left shoulder that I was in tears. I told a co-worker and she suggested that I try this massage therapy machine she would bring to work. I had to suffer all that night until the next day . . . I took half a Percocet to help relieve the pain.

The next day came and I was still in pain. Anyhow, my co-worker placed the machine's gel pads on my shoulder and immediately I was in tears from the comfort I was getting – from such a little device! She let me take the machine home for a week while she was away on travel, and I used it until the batteries ran out. It was so soothing. I will be purchasing one for myself in the near future. Oh what a relief!

– Germaine Drake; Decatur, Georgia

DEAR DR. HO:

I purchased Dr. Ho's Muscle Massage System several years ago from the Shopping Channel. I wanted relief from chronic headaches, neck and shoulder tension and pain due to arthritis. The system proved to be very effective and reduced pain almost immediately upon use. My husband has also used it for tennis elbow and plantar fasciitis. We have since purchased one for my father-in-law, who uses it for back and knee pain. Thanks for producing such a great convenient product that really works!

– Sherry Peressotti; Niagara Falls, Ontario

DEAR DR. HO:

I purchased Dr. Ho's Muscle Massage System a little over one year ago for my severe headaches and back pain. I first used it the day it arrived, and to my surprise the vigorous massager gave my muscles fast relief from many months of pain. I continue to use it as a regular routine. And when I happen to get a headache, I treat myself with Dr Ho's massage system and not pain medicine. I like that I can select different settings for massages, and that it requires only a few small batteries.

I rate Dr. Ho's Muscle Massage System as a must-have product! It has saved me hundreds of dollars on doctors and massage therapists. The product was also very easy to use – so simple my children have tried it. Thanks, Dr. Ho.

– Allyn Miller; Roscoe, Illinois

DEAR DR. HO:

Milliseconds after applying the gel pads to my weary shoulders, a deep feeling of relief penetrated my body. I have had severe shoulder pain for several years, but after using Dr. Ho's Muscle Massage System I feel complete relief. Words cannot describe how incredible I feel after using it. It is a truly wonderful experience.

And the product is a breeze to operate! Dr. Ho's Muscle Massage System is a terrific way to relax after a stressful day at the office or (in my case) on the tennis court. THANK YOU DR. HO! You are a miracle worker.

– Marissa Quimby; Roosterville, Idaho

DEAR DR. HO:

I have recently been diagnosed with fibromyalgia but I've been suffering from it for several years. Although I've found some relief from yoga, I hadn't had a completely pain-free day without medication for a very long time – until I bought Dr. Ho's Muscle Massage System last Thursday.

Since then I've used it every day, at least five times a day, on my neck, shoulders, middle back and lower back. All areas are feeling much better. I've gone most of today without any pain at all and I haven't taken any pain medication for days. The system is easy to use and discreet: I've worn it while working and no one realizes until I point it out.

I know it won't get rid of my condition, but Dr. Ho's Muscle Massage System is drastically improving how I feel each day. On a scale of one to ten, I rate it a twelve!

– M. Delain; Toronto, Ontario

DEAR DR. HO:

Amen to all of your positive testimonials and thank God for you! I was officially diagnosed with fibromyalgia and chronic fatigue syndrome three years ago, but had been suffering for years prior. I had to retire from my job due to carpal tunnel/supinator surgeries. The vertebrae of my neck is deteriorating, putting me in a lot of pain. I have spent thousands on doctors, medication, neurologists, massage therapists, chiropractors and acupuncturists, but can honestly say that I have NEVER *received such immediate, long-term relief as from your product.*

I saw you on the shopping club about three years ago and purchased your Muscle Massage System. I guess I was feeling better and put it away, forgetting all about it. Then the pain returned, and so did the doctors, but I remembered my Dr. Ho's Muscle Massage System. They want to operate on my neck, but I have been able to put it off (hopefully forever) because of your massage system. I wasn't able to travel before my introduction to your system, but now I can ride in a car and even in an airplane. If I do something that exasperates my muscles, I immediately put on my Muscle Massage System and get relief in about ten minutes.

I have told many people about your product wherever I travel. When I meet people in pain, I feel for them and want them to have the relief I experience. I've been wishing that you offered a unit with four pads, and see that you now do! I am planning on getting the new device and giving my former one to another "deserving soul."

Your product is so easy to take anywhere because it is so small and compact. Thank you, thank you, thank you! Sincerely,

– Ramona Bush; Bonita, California

Note from Dr. Ho: Because of all the valuable feedback I've received from people like Ramona, Dr. Ho's Muscle Massage System now comes with four electrode pads for a greater range of treatment options. We also offer large FlexTone pads to treat wider areas like the lower back and hip. You can order the system and supplementary attachments by simply calling us toll-free at 1-877-374-6669 (1-877-DRHONOW). Or visit our Web site at **www.drhonow.com**.

DEAR DR. HO:

I have suffered from "stress-induced" headaches and chronic neck and shoulder pain (from a car accident) for over fifteen years and have used MANY *forms of treatment. I even became addicted to pain medication as a result of always hurting. Using Dr. Ho's Muscle Massage System one to three times a day has provided heaven-sent relief that was virtually immediate. I bring it to work: nobody even knows I'm using it because it's invisible under clothes and so wonderfully easy to operate!*

I bought my first unit four years ago, recently purchased another – the Double Massage system – and am now ordering the large FlexTone pads. I can't wait to see how those feel on my lower back!

This product is a truly effective pain relief system with NO *side effects (except for the involuntary sighs of relief!) and I sincerely thank you, Dr. Ho, for making it available.*

– B.J. Young; Albuquerque, New Mexico

DEAR DR. HO:

I thought I should take the time to write you and let you know just how successful your product has been for me and my friends. I suffer from extremely painful muscle spasms in my shoulders, neck and middle back. I really did try everything – those big vibrating thumpers, massage, hot baths – and though they gave some temporary relief it was nothing compared to the everyday relief I get from your machine. Why, just on New Year's Eve this past year I had a crippling spasm in my mid-back which I was sure was going to land me in an emergency ward somewhere. I put the pads on and felt IMMEDIATE *relief. In one to two days the condition had eased up and disappeared altogether.*

I have suffered from muscle spasms for almost fifteen years, but achieved long-term relief after only two weeks of using the machine faithfully – one to two times a day. The best thing about the product is that I can take it anywhere; I travel a lot and it really helps to ease my tension daily. Its design is ideal, and I can't wait to try the new product you have out with the larger pads etc.

I have nothing bad to say about this product and I have even gone so far as to "sell" it to four friends by having them try mine. I even (you'll think I'm nuts!) urge people I see trying out the product at Dr. Ho kiosks to buy it immediately. It is one of the best investments I have ever made. Thanks.

– Robert Herriot; Toronto, Ontario

DEAR DR. HO:

I would just like to inform you of my wife's and my experience using the Dr. Ho's Muscle Massage System. She was involved in a car accident a couple of years ago and has since suffered from back and neck pain. Although physiotherapy and massage were beneficial, the benefits soon ran out. Furthermore, they were only available by appointment and required travel to a distant location.

With Dr. Ho, no appointment is necessary. Not only is it available 24/7, it is extremely helpful at providing relief from recurring pain. Relief comes with every application! Not only that, but the pain has subsided and doesn't return anywhere near as often.

I have started using the unit for left shoulder discomfort that I have been experiencing for the past six months. Dr. Ho provides instant relief. I especially like the second "chopping" setting and set it as high as I can tolerate. We now have to fight over the unit some days! Congratulations on this wonderful system.

– Gary and Mary Del Bianco; Concord, Ontario

PS: I would love to purchase the larger FlexTone pads, as I need to work on my abdominal muscles as part of an exercise program to help support my lower back.

> *Note from Dr. Ho: For all of you who want to order the larger Flextone pads, you can do so by simply calling us toll-free at 1-877-374-6669 (1-877-DRHONOW). Or visit our Web site at* **www.drhonow.com**.

DEAR DR. HO:

I have been meaning to send off an e-mail to you for over a year now, and have no idea why it has taken me so long. I purchased my Dr. Ho's Muscle Massage System in February 2001 while at the RV Show in Abbotsford, BC. At the time I was in severe pain and undergoing weekly chiropractic treatment for sciatic nerve pain in my right buttock and down my right leg as far as my ankle. I had been experiencing this pain for approximately six months and was not really getting much relief.

That day at the RV Show I was in a lot of pain and just could not resist the temptation of visiting the Dr. Ho booth where they were doing demos. I came away full of enthusiasm, clutching my newly purchased Dr. Ho unit. I used it extensively for the first two to three weeks and the relief was dramatic – I simply could not believe how the pain had lessened and how my outlook on life in general had improved. I kept up the treatment, but only every second or third day instead of every day – eventually I was able to scale back to weekly treatments – and for the most part the pain had disappeared.

The pain reoccurs from time to time, but I just go back onto regular Dr. Ho treatments and before long I am once again pain-free – unbelievable!!!! I just could not, and will not manage my pain without my Dr. Ho. My husband also finds my Dr. Ho to be a tremendous help when he gets headaches and extremely tight shoulder muscles.

On the subject of headaches and painful shoulder muscles, within a month of my Dr. Ho purchase I had already bought another unit from Batten Agencies in North Vancouver and mailed it to my daughter in England. She is an interior and architectural designer working long hours bent over a drawing board and working on a computer. Consequently, she was suffering from blinding headaches, neck pain and shoulder pain. She used her Dr. Ho as directed: the pain eased and the tension level in her neck improved dramatically.

After using the device for about a month, she realized with delight that her headaches were getting less frequent and she no longer needed to take her medication as often as she used to. She feels much better about herself and about life in general. Whereas before all she could do was stay home and lie down with her headache, she now often goes out in the evening to a show or to dinner. She still gets the odd headache but as soon as she feels one coming on, out comes the Dr. Ho! Her headaches never reach the intensity they did a year ago and she seldom feels the need to take any headache medication.

I thank you most sincerely for the tremendous relief Dr. Ho's Muscle Massage System has brought to me, my husband and most importantly to my precious daughter.

– Denise Johnson; Chilliwack, British Columbia

DEAR DR. HO:

I purchased Dr. Ho's Muscle Massage System about six months ago. I have suffered from arthritis in the knees on and off for about thirty years. During the last five years I have had trouble getting up from a sitting position without support. I began using your machine all over my body, never thinking that it could help my knees. But one day, I was able to stand right up without any pain or support, and I've been able to ever since.

I also have a bad circulation problem: I get cramps in my leg muscles whenever I walk very far or dance. Now I use Dr. Ho's Muscle Massage System before and after I go dancing or walking. I used to wake up screaming the morning after – in so much pain that I couldn't walk. I have been making progress on this problem for about a week and will let you know how it works. One thing I would like to see added to your machine is a band to hold the pads on the arms or legs. Thank you, Dr. Ho!

– H. Dalrymple; Coquitlam, British Columbia

Note from Dr. Ho: I find that in order to secure pads on skin with hair, such as the arms, or on awkward areas such as ankles, the pads are best held in place by an Ace bandage or the variety of bandage tape that sticks to itself and not to skin. You can find either in most pharmacies and convenience stores.

DEAR DR. HO:

Good afternoon. I wanted to let you know how much I enjoy using Dr. Ho's Muscle Massage System. Having been in a car accident several years ago, I have continuing problems with my lower back and neck. On the recommendation of my chiropractor Dr. Astrid Trim, I bought my first Dr. Ho about three years ago.

This unit is totally amazing! Many days, I would not be able to walk or turn my neck if I did not use Dr. Ho's Muscle Massage System. Thank you so much for making such a great product.

My daughter also suffers from back and neck pain so I gave her my Dr. Ho and she uses it faithfully. We had passed the single unit back and forth over the course of a year, but finally last week I bought my own – the new one is even better with four pads! I have just told someone in my office about it and she will be placing an order as well.

If you need someone to do any testimonials for Dr. Ho's Muscle Massage System, I would be more than happy to let the public know what a wonderful product it is. Once again, thank you for your great invention. It keeps me out of the chiropractor's office and saves me money!

– Judy McLellan; Mississauga, Ontario

DEAR DR. HO:

My name is Carol Long and I have fibromyalgia. I spent $2000 one year for chiropractic care but it only aggravated my problems. The only thing that has helped me at all is Dr. Ho's Muscle Massage System. I have now used it for two years and do not know what I would do without it – I just love it. Every day I thank you for coming up with this excellent product. Thank you!

– Carol Long

DEAR DR. HO:

I purchased my massage system about a year ago. My work predominantly takes place in front of a computer monitor all day, which causes a lot of strain on my neck and shoulders, often leading to headaches. When I first treated myself with Dr. Ho's Muscle Massage System, it instantly relieved the tension and thus relieved my headaches. Now I use it whenever the tightness in my muscles reappears. I've also shared it with my mother, who was experiencing the same type of muscle tension. She loves it just as much as I do. Sometimes we fight over who will use it first! Thank you, Dr. Ho.

– Andrea McClendon; Kapolei, Hawaii

DEAR DR. HO:

I would just like to praise the effectiveness of your wonderful machine. I am an artist who engraves jewellery for a living, but was diagnosed with rotator cuff syndrome caused by years of poor posture on the job. I damaged a lot of the muscles and tissues in my back and shoulders. Before purchasing and applying Dr. Ho's Muscle Massage System I could not sleep at night, nor lift my arms over my shoulders. I began using Dr. Ho every day for about a month and it has worked wonders: I've felt great improvement, and movement without pain has become possible for me again. I can now reach over my head without any pain! Thanks Dr. Ho for this wonderful device.

From a happy customer,

– Ann Mellish; Nanaimo, British Columbia

DEAR DR. HO:

I have had Dr. Ho's Muscle Massage System for a couple of years and could not be without it. Before I purchased your machine, my lower back pain was so bad that upon waking some mornings I could not get up. Now, I keep the machine right beside my bed and when I awake I put it on for twenty minutes – then I can face the day.

My chiropractor is extremely impressed with the improvement of my back: he told me it has not been this good for years! I have had other injuries as well, but this little machine fixes all my problems. It's the first item I pack in my suitcase whenever I go anywhere. Thank you Dr. Ho for making my life easier.

– Linda Jones; Saskatoon, Saskatchewan

These are but a few out of many hundreds of positive letters I've received since developing the system. If you have *Dr. Ho's Muscle Massage System*, I truly hope that you will write me and share your experiences with the device. I am always interested in how people respond to **TENS** therapy; I use people's comments to continually improve the product, its attachments and its implementation to best reduce and eliminate pain.

I look forward to hearing from you!

Index